Drug Treatment in Old Age Psychiatry

Cornelius Katona MD FRCPsych

Professor of Psychiatry of the Elderly, Department of Psychiatry and Behavioural Sciences, University College London, London

Gill Livingston MD FRCPsych

Reader in Psychiatry of Older People, Department of Psychiatry and Behavioural Sciences, University College London, London

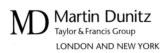

Martin Dunitz
Taylor & Francis Group
LONDON AND NEW YORK

D0317144

© 2003 Martin Dunitz, an imprint of Taylor & Francis

First published in the United Kingdom in 2003
by Martin Dunitz, an imprint of Taylor and Francis, 11 New Fetter Lane,
London EC4P 4EE

Tel.: +44 (0) 20 7583 9855
Fax. +44 (0) 20 7842 2298
E-mail: info@dunitz.co.uk
Website: http://www.dunitz.co.uk

Although every effort has been made to ensure that all owners of copyright material have been acknowledged in this publication, we would be glad to acknowledge in subsequent reprints or editions any omissions brought to our attention.

Although every effort has been made to ensure that drug doses and other information are presented accurately in this publication, the ultimate responsibility rests with the prescribing physician. Neither the publishers nor the authors can be held responsible for errors or for any consequences arising from the use of information contained herein. For detailed prescribing information or instructions on the use of any product or procedure discussed herein, please consult the prescribing information or instructional material issued by the manufacturer.

A CIP record for this book is available from the British Library.

ISBN 1 84184 225 7

Distributed in the USA by
Fulfilment Center
Taylor & Francis
10650 Tobben Drive
Independence, KY 41051, USA
Toll Free Tel.: +1 800 634 7064
E-mail: taylorandfrancis@thomsonlearning.com

Distributed in Canada by
Taylor & Francis
74 Rolark Drive
Scarborough, Ontario M1R 4G2, Canada
Toll Free Tel.: +1 877 226 2237
E-mail: tal_fran@istar.ca

Distributed in the rest of the world by
Thomson Publishing Services
Cheriton House
North Way
Andover, Hampshire SP10 5BE, UK
Tel.: +44 (0)1264 332424
E-mail: salesorder.tandf@thomsonpublishingservices.co.uk

Composition by Wearset Ltd, Boldon, Tyne and Wear

Printed and bound in Great Britain by The Cromwell Press, Trowbridge.

Contents

Foreword

In *Drug Treatment in Old Age Psychiatry*, Katona and Livingston have bridged what for many years has been a significant gap in the information-rich world of psychopharmacology.

Psychopharmacology books are many but very few deal with the elderly and those which do are designed for specialist old age psychiatrists which while valuable, do not assist the multi-disciplinary team which is the backbone of all mental health and medical services designed to serve older people with mental disorders.

This is a clinically relevant, succinct, user-friendly text based on available evidence (little it may be in some areas) to provide a solid framework to understand, appreciate and apply the art and science of drug treatment to the older person with mental disorders. The primary care physician, general physician, community-based and inpatient nurses, allied health professionals, as well as medical undergraduates will benefit from this book being available for quick reference.

To this end the 'boxes' which summarizes the essential issues will, at a glance, assist in the practice level as well as in developing teaching material.

The chapters on Co-morbid depression in the context of other illnesses, Treatment of behavioural and psychological symptoms of dementia (BPSD), Delirium, and Psychotropics in drug interaction are most up-to-date and very useful. These are subjects not often and not succinctly covered by many books on psychopharmacotherapy, and this reflects the very 'hands-on' clinical practice of the two authors who are the clinician's clinicians.

The field of old age psychiatry, community practice and primary care owe Katona and Livingston a great thank you for their perspicacity in conceptualizing and delivery of this text, and to Martin Dunitz for publishing this in a format which is a model for clinically useful small reference books for clinicians.

Edmond Chiu AM
Professor, Academic Unit for Psychiatry of Old Age
University of Melbourne
Australia

Preface

Nowhere is it more important to get psychotropic drug prescribing 'right' than in old age psychiatry practice, given the increased vulnerability of older people to adverse drug effects and to dangerous interactions. Although there are many excellent textbooks dealing with psychiatric drug prescribing in general and with old age psychiatry, there is a remarkable lack of summary texts addressing the specific issues of psychotropic drug prescribing for older people.

We have attempted to produce a short, portable and practical book that should be helpful to psychiatrists (including those in training), to pharmacists and to physicians in medicine for older people. It should also be useful for nurses and psychologists working with older people because they are becoming increasingly involved in the practicalities of drug administration.

We have attempted to review the literature systematically and hope that the summary text we have produced is an accurate and up-to-date reflection of the current evidence base. In the interests of brevity, legibility and portability, we have chosen not to cite all the hundreds of references we have summarized. We have, however, appended a brief list of systematic reviews and more general papers and textbooks, which we hope will help guide readers who require more detailed information.

Writing the book has made us intensely aware that good prescribing is an art as well as a science. Prescribers need to be aware of the range of available drugs, their characteristics and limitations, and the problems commonly encountered in their use. Equally important, they need to take into account the individual characteristics, wishes and knowledge of the patients involved and their families. We hope that, by summarizing the core knowledge currently available, this book will encourage good and individualized practice.

Cornelius Katona
Gill Livingston

chapter 1

Practicalities of drug treatment in old age

Adherence and compliance: just keep taking the tablets

The scale of the problem

All tablets are ineffective if not taken. Adherence is often poor, with between 30% and 68% of patients discontinuing antidepressants and a further third taking too few, too many or irregularly. Patients who do not recover from depression are often those who have discontinued or never taken their medication.

Ways to increase adherence

The research into improving adherence is comparatively recent in its development. Factors identified as important in non-adherence for all age groups include patient attitudes, social circumstances, side effects of medication and the quality of the patient–doctor relationship. It is well established in the literature that a complex interplay of factors may be involved in an individual's non-adherence to antidepressants. However, such awareness has not yet permeated the majority of research into adherence interventions. A review of 17 studies in younger adults found that 15 were focused on patient education. (Pampallona et al, 2002) Although such education improves patients' knowledge, several studies have failed to demonstrate the translation of this into improved adherence or better outcome. Knowledge is not necessarily power.

The two exceptions to didactic information-based approaches to increasing adherence included some form of exploration of potential obstacles to adherence from a patient's perspective. A trial of a cognitive–behavioural intervention combined with psychoeducation (compliance therapy) was compared with non-specific counselling for patients with psychosis on acute psychiatric admissions wards. This resulted in the development of a manual for use in this patient group. The second, published in 1999, was a trial of antidepressant drug counselling conducted by nurses in primary care compared with drug information leaflets. Both study interventions improved adherence in comparison to their control groups.

The literature on adherence interventions for the older population is fairly sparse. Only one small non-randomized study has specifically addressed the use of antidepressants in elderly people. It suggested that one-off family therapy sessions improve adherence.

Several other strategies have been explored for use with a variety of medical interventions in older people. Efforts to improve adherence with one-off treatments, using written educational material, have had mixed results; one study demonstrated increased uptake of influenza immunization with this method whereas another failed to demonstrate such an effect for colorectal cancer screening. For longer-term treatments, two patient education programmes conducted by pharmacists have shown a positive impact on adherence. A further study failed to demonstrate any benefit from adding a medication card to pharmacist-led patient education. It is of note, however, that most of the research on older people focuses on the mechanics of medication delivery, such as the successful use of calendar blister packs. This move away from emphasis on cognitive aspects of adherence may in part reflect stereotyping of older people as cognitively impaired.

The literature on adherence for both younger and older people suggests that patients often do an informal cost–benefit analysis to decide whether to take medication. This has been formalized in what is known as the health belief model (see *Box 1* which lists the areas considered).

Non-adherence to antidepressants

Factors associated with non-adherence to antidepressants are lack of

Box 1   Health belief model.

- Perceived threat of illness
- Internal cues to action, e.g. pain
- External cues to action, e.g. GP advice
- Perceived benefits of treatment
- Perceived costs of treatment

education about the medication from the prescriber, and worry about experience of side effects. Tackling these factors may help ensure that people take their medication (*Box 2*). Our group has recently developed a form of concordance therapy for older people with depression combining elements of psychoeducation, motivation therapy and cognitive–behavioural therapy.

Box 2   Factors associated with increased adherence to antidepressants.

- Prescribing tablets with fewer side effects
- Discussing the tablets with and educating the patient about the tablets
- Finding out and addressing patient's worries about side effects.

Non-adherence to anti-psychotics

Patients often do not take anti-psychotic medication (*Box 3*). The reasons may be similar to those mentioned above, e.g. unacceptable side effects. There may be additional factors; one study of younger people

Box 3   Factors associated with adherence to anti-psychotics.

- Less severe psychotic symptoms
- Good sense of relation to self or others
- Low agreement regarding purpose of treatment

has found that the most important predictor for not taking the tablets in this population was severity of psychotic symptoms. This may be related to disorganization, apathy or a lack of insight into having an illness.

Dementia and non-adherence (*Box 4*)

Non-adherence in dementia may be related to the inability to remember whether the tablets have been taken. There is also a marked similarity to the psychotic illnesses in that patients may not believe that they are ill, have difficulty in organizing themselves to take the tablets or are apathetic. People with dementia may benefit from some of the general strategies discussed in *Box 5* such as a dosset box. Frequently, if the dementia is more than very mild, the patients need supervision because they will have difficulty learning to use a dosset box or finding it. Most supervision is done by the family at home or by paid carers if a person is institutionalized. Those people who live alone with care packages can be reminded by the carers to take their medication, but the carers are not

Box 4   Reasons for non-adherence in dementia.

- Inability to remember whether tablets have been taken
- Patients believe that they are well
- Patients have difficulty organizing themselves to take the tablets
- Apathy

Box 5   Strategies for managing general difficulties in taking medication.

- Prescriber should ensure that regimen is as simple as possible
- Prescriber should review medication regularly to ensure that the patient is not on unnecessary tablets
- Dosset box
- Pharmacy-filled, dated, individualized containers
- Liquid medication
- Non-childproof containers

allowed to sort it out. This group of people will therefore require a pharmacist, district nurse or member of the family to put the medication into special packaging, a dosset box or other container.

Difficulties in taking medication: general problems in older people (*Box 6*)

We have discussed the reasons why people may choose not to take medication. In addition to these problems, older people more commonly have specific difficulties in taking medication related to specific or multiple morbidities. The difficulties may be related to a particular psychiatric problem such as dementia or psychosis and these are discussed above. There may also be difficulties related to physical illnesses, such as problems in swallowing or difficulty in getting the tablets out of the container. People with multiple morbidities may have very complex medication regimens which are difficult to follow even in those who are motivated to do so, cognitively intact and organized. Since many older patients with multiple illnesses are depressed or have dementia, these may be additional complications.

Box 6   Factors associated with general difficulty in taking tablets.

- Forgetting to take the tablets
- Difficulty in swallowing
- Difficulty in getting the tablets out of the container
- Complex medication regimens

Strategies for tackling general problems in taking tablets (see *Box 5*)

Many complex medication regimens do not need to be as difficult. It is the duty of the prescriber to ensure that the regimen is as simple as possible, e.g. by ensuring that medication is not prescribed twice a day if it can be taken on a once-daily basis. Many patients have more and more tablets added without any being removed. It is also essential that prescribing doctors review medication regularly to ensure that the patient is not on unnecessary tablets. Patients who have difficulties in accessing drugs, e.g. because of muscular weakness or arthritis, may benefit from a more easily accessible container such as a dosset box or ticking the box on prescription that specifies non-childproof containers. Dosset boxes can also be very useful to sort out complex medication regimens, although they require to be filled manually. This may sometimes be done by relatives or district nurses.

An easier alternative may be the packaging service offered by most community pharmacists where all of a patient's drugs are dispensed in an individualized pack that is labelled with the times and days of the week. Reviewing the packaging and number of tablets may help patients who have a degree of difficulty in swallowing. Some will require their medication in liquid form and this may not be readily available and may have to be specially made.

Paradoxically, patients who can swallow nothing may have no difficulty with tablets. They usually require nutrition through a percutaneous endoscopic gastrostomy (PEG) and medication can be given in the same way.

chapter 2

Depression

Definition and symptoms

Depression is common and disabling in old age, particularly in people who have co-morbid physical illness or are in institutional care. It is associated with high costs for health care and social care. Despite this, it is often missed, ignored or not managed adequately. Patients present when they need help but often they do not complain of low mood. This is partly a consequence of widely held 'ageist' assumptions that depression is intrinsic to the ageing process, and that treatment is inappropriate, excessively risky or unlikely to be effective. These assumptions are demonstrably untrue: most older people are not clinically depressed (despite their increased risk of loss and adversity); depression does not increase in prevalence with age and those who are depressed respond as well to the range of pharmacological and psychological treatment as do younger depressed patients.

Clinical features

Depression often presents in a less typical fashion in old age. The clinical features of depressive disorder may also be complicated by coexisting medical problems and/or cognitive impairment. This clearly has implications for the under- or misdiagnosis of depression in elderly people. Older patients tend to have an increase in somatic complaints, sleep disturbance (initial insomnia) and agitation. Two main symptom clusters have been demonstrated: 'affective suffering', which includes low mood, tearfulness and the wish to die; and a 'motivational' cluster comprising loss of interest, poor concentration and lack of enjoyment (*Box 7*). Some depressive symptomatology is often found in older individuals who do *not* have frank depressive illness. The psychological symptoms most frequently elicited in such people include dysphoria, sleep disturbance, thoughts of death, anergy, impaired concentration, agitation and retardation.

Box 7   Symptom clusters in depression in elderly people.

Affective suffering
Low mood
Tearfulness
The wish to die

Motivational cluster
Loss of interest
Poor concentration
Lack of enjoyment

Age-related differences in symptom patterns have been reported in elderly people. Items relating to low self-esteem were more common in the 'young old', whereas the presence of hypochondriasis was positively correlated with age. Individuals whose first episode of depression occurred in late life are more likely to display cognitive impairment, although psychotic features occur less often. However, the latter finding may be a reflection of the greater average age (and therefore greater vulnerability to dementia) of those in the group with late first onset. Symptom patterns in depressed older people have been found to differ by sex. Depressed mood, guilt, anxiety and diurnal mood variation were found to be more common in women with depression than in men with depression.

Prevalence and associates of depression

Older individuals in the community appear to have a lower prevalence of *major* depression (as defined within the DSM [*Diagnostic and Statistical Manual of Mental Disorders*] system) than their younger counterparts whereas the prevalence of dysthymia (chronic mild depression) may be much higher. This probably reflects the differences in typical clinical features discussed above. Two recent comprehensive reviews (mainly of studies using interview schedules and diagnostic criteria designed specifically for use in older people) reported average prevalence rates of 13.5% and 12.3%. Most of the studies reviewed found rates in women nearly twice as high as in men.

The prevalence of depressive illness appears to be higher among those elderly people who attend their general practitioner (GP). Rates as high as 34% have been reported. Frequent attendance at the GP surgery may be a 'marker' of increased likelihood of depression. Similarly, the prevalence of depressive disorders among elderly people in long-term institutional care is in excess of 20%. In hospitalized elderly people, the prevalence of depression rises further, with a reported range between 12% and 45%.

Depression is more common in physically ill than in healthy older people. As physical illness and depression often both present with physical features (such as sleep disturbance, loss of appetite and pain), the use of screening tests that use biological symptoms can lead to false positives. The main risk factors for depression appear to be the severity of physical illness, the degree of disability, coexisting cognitive impairment and a positive past psychiatric history. Physical disability seems to be particularly strongly associated with depression in insitutional settings. Depression in older medical patients frequently becomes chronic, and in turn appears to have an adverse effect on the physical prognosis, especially in terms of likelihood of successful rehabilitation. In addition, older medical patients with depression consume more healthcare resources, have longer admissions and a higher mortality, and are more likely to be transferred to residential care. However, depression in older medical patients is frequently overlooked by medical staff, despite high rates of depressive symptomatology. Its detection may be facilitated by simple screening tests.

The most striking vulnerability factors for depression identified in community surveys are social, including poverty, bereavement and social isolation. Life events often precipitate depression in old age. Several community studies have emphasized the importance of the concept of loss in understanding the depression of old age. The availability of a confidant(e) may act as a buffer against such loss-related depression, particularly in women. Those individuals who are separated, divorced or widowed exhibit more depressive illness than single or married individuals. Several studies have found that being a caregiver for someone with dementia or depression is associated with an increased risk of depression in the caregiver; this is particularly marked in women, in spouse caregivers, where the pre-morbid relationship was poor and where there are prominent behavioural problems such as aggression.

The management of depression in old age

Depression is underdetected and undertreated

Only a small minority of older patients with depression receive treatment. A community study found that only 13% of those with depression were being treated with antidepressants; at follow-up the figure remained virtually the same at 14%. Similarly, only 10% of patients with depression identified by consecutive primary care attenders were receiving treatment for depression, although in 95% of cases their GPs were able to identify them as depressed. Even when older people *are* prescribed antidepressants, the doses given are frequently subtherapeutic.

There are several possible reasons for this underprescribing (*Box 8*). Depression in older patients may be missed owing to its frequent manifestation as symptoms not immediately identified as depressive, such as anxiety or somatic complaints. It may also not be diagnosed if the symptoms displayed are viewed as a 'normal' response to ageing, physical impairment or living alone. Doctors may be reluctant to prescribe medication to older patients because of concerns about adverse effects and lack of knowledge about the different side effects of the various agents; this may account for the common prescription of medication at subtherapeutic doses. As a result, GPs may conceptualize depression in old age as a legitimate and unavoidable consequence of ageing and associated adversity, which is recognizable but not seen as treatable.

Box 8 Reasons for undertreatment of depression in old age.

- Prominent anxiety or somatic complaints
- Symptoms seen as 'normal' response to:
  - ageing
  - physical impairment
  - living alone
- Depression seen as legitimate consequence of ageing and adversity
- Lack of knowledge about drug side effects in old age
- Fear of adverse effects

Goals of treatment of depression (Box 9 and Figure 1)

Depression is associated with suicide and the first responsibility of the clinician is to assess the risk of suicide and to prevent suicide with appropriate management. The next aim is to achieve a significant reduction in symptom severity. This should not, however, be seen as

---

Box 9 Goals of treatment of depression.

- Assessment of risk of suicide
- Prevention of suicide
- Reduction in symptoms
- Remission of symptoms
- Prevention of relapse
- Prevention of recurrence
- Restoration of social functioning
  - interpersonal relationships
  - self-care

adequate; a more important goal within the acute treatment phase is full remission of symptoms – which is achieved much less often than symptom reduction.

As depression is a chronic and recurring illness, the goals of treatment are alleviation of symptoms leading not only to eventual remission but also to preventing relapse (during the period of recovery) and recurrence (after a period of being well). These phases are illustrated in *Figure 1*. This means that continuation treatment is essential after alleviation of symptoms and that maintenance treatment should be considered to prevent recurrence. Depression is associated with a decrease in social functioning, interpersonal relationships and self-care. Restoration of functioning is another important goal of treatment.

Acute treatment

Drug trials usually use a 50% reduction in the depression severity scale as a measure of response, i.e. 50% reduction in the score on the Hamilton Scale. This indicates that the patient has improved but not necessarily that

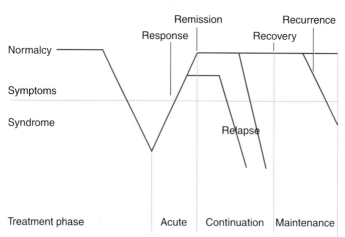

Figure 1 *Graphic representation of the phases of treatment for depressive disorder (after Frank et al 1991).*

he or she is well. Other drug trials use the end-point of 'remission', which is achieved only when the patient is no longer depressed according to usual criteria used to diagnose depression or has only negligible depressive symptoms (< 7 on the Hamilton Scale). Clinically the goal of treatment should be remission rather than simply improvement, not only because this will reduce individual suffering but also because incompletely treated depression is associated with a much higher rate of recurrence. Even with the best treatment, antidepressant monotherapy is not always successful. It is therefore important to have a rational strategy about how to manage those who are resistant to initial treatment. This is discussed below.

Difficulties in prescribing antidepressants for older adults

Antidepressants are undeniably more hazardous in old age, because of age-related pharmacokinetic changes and the high frequency in older people of coexistent medical problems and co-administered drugs that may interact adversely with antidepressants. Some of the adverse effects of antidepressants, particularly falls, are potentially much more serious in old age.

Age-related reductions in creatinine clearance, hepatic blood flow and plasma protein levels in older patients typically result in higher plasma levels of many drugs, including tricyclic antidepressants (TCAs). This is less so for new antidepressants and often no dose adjustment is necessary. The elimination half-life of some selective serotonin re-uptake inhibitors (SSRIs) such as paroxetine and citalopram is significantly increased in old age; this is much less marked for other SSRIs (fluoxetine or fluvoxamine). It must, however, be borne in mind that there is considerable variability in drug absorption, distribution, metabolism and excretion between individuals caused, for example, by genetically determined differences in cytochrome P450 isoenzyme levels.

The same side effects may be more hazardous in older compared with younger adults. Both TCAs and monoamine oxidase inhibitors (MAOIs) have a propensity to produce adverse effects that are likely to be more dangerous in older patients. These include anticholinergic, antihistaminic and anti-adrenergic effects. Vulnerability to falls relates mainly to the potency of older TCAs, which act as α_1-adrenergic receptor blockers which thereby aggravate postural hypotension. An increase in falls and fractures is perhaps the most hazardous consequence of these. In addition, MAOIs require dietary restriction, and TCAs may have a quinidine-like effect and cause tachycardia and prolongation of the Q–T interval. The anticholinergic side effects can lead to urinary retention, constipation and glaucoma. Not all antidepressants within a class have identical side effects, e.g. nortriptyline causes relatively little postural hypotension and is widely used in old age psychiatry practice in the USA, and lofepramine is relatively free of anticholinergic side effects, causes little cognitive impairment and is very safe in overdose. Much of the data about efficacy has to be extrapolated from work that includes very few or no older people. There are few trials that are exclusively in older people and they tend to have relatively low numbers (see below). In particular few data are available on the pure noradrenaline re-uptake inhibitor (NARI) reboxetine (which is not at present recommended for use in older people) and the serotonin (5-hydroxytryptamine or 5HT) antagonist SSRI nefazodone.

Antidepressant-induced hyponatraemia caused by inappropriate antidiuretic hormone secretion occurs almost exclusively in older people. It is a rare but potentially serious complication that can lead to acute confusion and then to seizures. Older patients with co-morbid medical disorders are the group at risk of this relatively rare complication.

In addition to the age-related pharmacological differences outlined above, older people are more likely to have significant physical and/or cognitive co-morbidity which antidepressant drugs may affect adversely.

Interaction with other medication is a more frequent problem as patients age. This is considered in more detail below.

General factors relating to choice of antidepressant in older people

Several factors (*Box 10*) should be taken into account when choosing an antidepressant. They will vary with individual patients. There is no one drug or class of drug that will suit all older patients and the prescription should be tailored to the individual. Some patients may have marked and health-threatening weight loss. Mirtazapine is particularly helpful in stimulating weight gain. Other patients may have distressing sleep disturbance or hypersomnia, and the effect of a drug on sleep should be considered. Mirtazapine may, again, be particularly useful in this context.

There may be a prior history of response or otherwise to a particular drug or class; this may help predict efficacy in the present episode. There may also be a history of tolerance or intolerance to a particular drug. Drug safety is paramount. Careful note needs to be taken of other prescribed (or over-the-counter) preparations that the patient is taking in terms of possible adverse interactions. Equally important, a patient may have one or more particular medical condition that could be exacerbated by a particular drug. TCAs may, for example, trigger urinary retention in the context of benign prostatic hyperplasia. Lethality in overdose is a very important consideration in patients thought to be at risk of suicide. Some TCAs (amitriptyline, dothiepin, desipramine) are particularly hazardous in this context. The cost of antidepressants varies enormously, with older drugs and those available generically being much cheaper.

Categories of antidepressant available
The categories of antidepressant available are summarized in *Table 1*: the TCAs, SSRIs, the MAOIs, the reversal inhibitors of MAO-A (RIMAs), and atypical antidepressants such as the serotonin and noradrenaline

---

Box 10   Factors to be considered in choosing an antidepressant.

- Efficacy
- Speed of onset
- Profile of symptoms
- Ease of administration
- Tolerability
- Safety
- Interactions
- Lethality in overdose
- Cost

reuptake inhibitor (SNRI) venlafaxine, the noradrenaline reuptake inhibitor (NARI) reboxetine, the noradrenaline and specific serotonin antidepressant (NASSA) mirtazapine, and others such as mianserin and trazodone. The recommended starting and maintenance doses and the significant adverse effects and contraindications of antidepressant drugs in older people are shown in *Table 1*. *Table 2* shows the mode of action and important receptor interactions and recommended daily doses of antidepressants in older people.

Efficacy of antidepressants

Conclusions from drug trials should be tempered with the awareness that trial samples are somewhat unrepresentative of clinical populations. Controlled trials of tricyclic and newer antidepressant drugs have consistently demonstrated response rates of 50–60% in older people, compared with 25% for placebo.

In 'real-life' practice response rates are lower. Newer antidepressants may, because of their better side-effect and safety profile, have greater advantage than is apparent in the 'super-fit, super-depressed' individuals who are eligible for clinical trials. There is some evidence that antidepressants may take as long as 10–12 weeks to show clinical improvement in older people.

There is a dearth of placebo-controlled trials of newer drugs in particular, with the exception of citalopram (Nyth et al, 1992), fluoxetine (Tollefson et al, 1995; Wakelin, 1986) and moclobemide (Nair et al, 1995). Head-to-head comparisons between newer and older antidepressants, however, suggest similar efficacy rates for most drugs, although with some important exceptions. The studies are reviewed in detail below.

Systematic reviews of antidepressants

A recent meta-analysis of controlled trials of the main classes of antidepressant drugs (TCAs, SSRIs, RIMAs and atypical antidepressants) found all to be superior to placebo, but did not reveal significant differences between classes. This may in part reflect the reduced statistical power of such meta-analyses as well as the blurring of differences between drugs within a class.

Table 1 Classes of antidepressants, recommended doses and significant side effects in older patients.

Antidepressant class	Examples	Starting dose (mg/day)	Maintenance dose (mg/day)	Adverse effects	Contraindications
TCA	Amitriptyline	25	100–150	Confusion, blurred vision constipation, urinary retention, orthostatic hypotension, cardiac arrhythmias, reduced seizure threshold, sedation (more with amitriptyline and trimipramine; less with lofepramine)	Prostatism, narrow angle glaucoma, post-myocardial infarction, heart block
	Imipramine	10	75–150		
	Nortiptyline	20	20–150		
	Lofepramine	70	140–210		
	Dothiepin	75	75–150		
	Desipramine	75	75–150		
	Clomipramine	10	50–150		
	Trimipramine	75	75–150		
SSRI	Fluoxetine	10–20	20–40	Nausea (most common with fluvoxamine), diarrhoea, headache, agitation (particularly fluoxetine) sedation, decrease of seizure threshold Weight loss and rash with fluoxetine	MAOI
	Citalopram	10–20	20–40		
	Paroxetine	10–20	20–40		
	Fluvoxamine	100	100–300		
	Sertraline	50	50–100		

Table 1 continued

Antidepressant class	Examples	Starting dose (mg/day)	Maintenance dose (mg/day)	Adverse effects	Contraindications
				Withdrawal syndrome with anxiety and dizziness (especially with paroxetine) Decreased libido and anorgasmia Occasionally hyponatraemia Occasionally extra pyramidal side effects	
MAOI	Phenelzine Tranylcypromine Isocarboxazid	15 10 30 (for up to 6 weeks	15-45 10-30 10-20	Confusion, weight gain, hypotension, constipation, urinary retention, sedation hepatotoxicity, oedema, leukopenia, psychosis, hypertensive crisis unless tyramine-containing foods avoided	Cardiovascular disease, phaeochromocytoma, liver disease, diabetes

Table 1 *continued*

Antidepressant class	Examples	Starting dose (mg/day)	Maintenance dose (mg/day)	Adverse effects	Contraindications
RIMA	Moclobemide	150	150–600	Agitation, insomnia somnolence,	MAOIs; hepatic or renal impairment (use lower doses)
SNRI	Venlafaxine	37.5	75–150	nausea, headache, dry mouth, rash (if drug related mandates cessation of drug) hypertension, sexual dysfunction, withdrawal syndrome	
NASSA	Mirtazapine	15	15–45	Sedation, weight gain, rarely blood dyscrasias, convulsions, myoclonus, oedema	
Atypical	Mianserin	30	30–90	Sedation, aplastic anaemia, agitation, priapism	
	Trazodone	100	300	Sedation, cardiotoxicity, hypotension	
	Nefazodone	100	200–400		

MAOI, monoamine oxidase inhibitor; NASSA, noradrenaline and specific serotonin antidepressant; RIMA, reversible inhibitor of MAO-A; SNRI, serotonin and noradrenaline reuptake inhibitor; SSRI, selective serotonin reuptake inhibitor; TCA, tricyclic antidepressant.

Table 2 Mode of action, receptor interaction and average daily dose of the main antidepressants.

Drug	Main mode of action	Anti-cholinergic	Anti-histaminic	α_1-Adrenergic blocking
Amitriptyline	NE++ 5HT+	++++	++++	++++
Imipramine	NE++ 5HT+	+++	++	+++
Nortripyline	NE++ 5HT+	+++	++	++
Dothiepin (dosulepin)	NE++ 5HT+	+++	++	++
Mianserin	α_2	0/+	+++	0/+
Lofepramine	NE++ 5HT+	+	+	+
Trazodone	$5HT_2$	0	+++	+
Fluvoxamine	5HT	0/+	0/+	0
Sertraline	5HT	0/+	0	0
Fluoxetine	5HT	0/+	0	0
Paroxetine	5HT	0/+	0	0
Citalopram	5HT	0/+	0	0
Phenelzine	Monoamine oxidase inhibition (non-reversible)	0/+	0	++
Moclobemide	MAO	0/+	0	0
Venlafaxine	NE+ 5HT++ α_2	0/+	0	0/+
Mirtazapine	$5HT_2$	0	++	0
Nefazodone	$5HT_2$	0	+	+

5HT, serotonin re-uptake inhibition; NE, norepinephrine (noradrenaline) re-uptake inhibition; DA, dopamine re-uptake inhibition; α_2, antagonism at the presynaptic α_2-receptor; +/++, indicates magnitude of side effect.

The Cochrane review of randomized placebo-controlled trials of anti-depressant treatment in people aged 60 years or more excluded studies that included people with dementia. They found 11 trials of TCAs (which they considered together), two trials of fluoxetine (the only SSRI considered), two of MAOIs and three of other drugs (classifieds as atypicals and also considered as a single class). TCAs, MAOIs and fluoxetine were efficacious when compared with placebo, and efficacy was apparent in all settings examined (community, hospital and institutions).

It is difficult to extrapolate the likely clinical response in individual patients from mean change statistics that are often quoted in papers, or from meta-analyses of classes of drug rather than individual drugs. The concept of 'number needed to treat' (NNT) has been suggested as useful in rendering randomized controlled trial (RCT) data meaningful for clinical decision-making, because it conveys both statistical and clinical information intelligibly. The NNT is the number of patients who need to be treated with the treatment in question, compared with another treatment (often placebo), for one patient to gain a specified benefit, e.g. if the NNT was three for antidepressant drug A, this would mean that you need to treat three older depressed people with drug A, for the duration of the trial specified, for one *more* of them to respond to A than the comparator (whether it was drug or placebo). The lower the NNT, the greater the advantage of the drug. Calculating NNTs enables a direct method of comparing different trials and provides a global outcome measure.

Where the clinical outcome being evaluated is adverse (e.g. side effects) the same calculation can generate a 'number needed to harm' (NNH). We recently completed a meta-analysis of antidepressant treatment in older people using NNTs. The results are summarized in *Tables 3–5* and increase the evidence base available to make clinical decisions about choice of antidepressant for older people.

The inclusion criteria were as follows:

- The study was double blinded, randomized and controlled.
- Efficacy measures, numbers of patients in each group and percentage of responders were reported.
- Diagnosis of major depressive disorder or unipolar depression used defined criteria.

Table 3 Numbers needed to treat for response rates in placebo-controlled antidepressant trials in old age.

Authors	Drug	N (active)	N (placebo)	Percentage response active	Percentage response placebo	Measure	NNT	95% CI
Cohn et al (1984)	Imipramine	21	21	82.0	45.0	CGI improved	3	2–10
Wakelin (1986)	Imipramine	29	14	65.0	25.0	CGI much improved	3	1–10
Merideth et al (1984)	Imipramine	14	15	64.3	20.0	CGI improved	2	1–8
Katz et al (1990)	Nortriptyline	12	11	58.3	9.1	HAMD very much improved	2	1–6
Katz et al (1990)	Nortriptyline	12	11	83.3	18.2	HAMD improved	1	1–2
Nair et al (1995)	Nortriptyline	38	35	31.6	8.6	HAMD < 10	5	2–28
Cohn et al (1984)	Nomifensine	21	21	82.0	45.0	CGI improved	3	2–10
Merideth et al (1984)	Nomifensine	19	15	78.9	20.0	CGI improved	2	1–3

Table 3 *continued*

Authors	Drug	N (active)	N (placebo)	Percentage response active	Percentage response placebo	Measure	NNT	95% CI
Nyth et al (1992)	Citalopram	60	34	53.0	28.0	MADRS < 50%	4	2–21
Nyth et al (1992)	Citalopram	60	34	60.0	24.0	CGI improvement	3	2–6
Nyth et al (1992)	Citalopram	60	34	70.0	47.0	CGI normal to mildly ill	4	2–32
Eli Lilly (1993)	Fluoxetine	29	41	31.0	34.1	HAMD	32	4–∞
Tollefson et al (1995)	Fluoxetine	335	336	43.9	31.6	HAMD response	8	5–20
Tollefson et al (1995)	Fluoxetine	335	336	31.6	18.6	HAMD remission	8	5–15
Wakelin (1986)	Fluvoxamine	33	14	79.0	25.0	CGI much improved	2	1–4
Nair et al (1995)	Moclobemide	36	35	22.2	8.6	HAMD < 10	7	3–∞

95% CI, 95% confidence interval/ N, number; NNT, number needed to treat; HAMD, Hamilton Depression Rating Scale; MADRS, Montgomery Asberg Depression Rating Scale; CGI, clinical global impression.

Table 4 Numbers needed to treat for head-to-head comparisons of antidepressant therapies.

Authors	Drugs	N (drug 1)	N (drug 2)	Measure	Percentage response drug 1	Percentage response drug 2	NNT	95% CI
Cohn et al (1990)	Ser/Ami	161	80	50% reduction HAMD	69.4	62.5	14 (Ser)	5–∞
Cohn et al	Ser/Ami	161	80	CGI improvement	79.5	73.4	16 (Ser)	6–∞
Finkel et al (1999)	Ser/Flx	42	33	HAMD response	58.5	42.4	6 (Ser)	3–∞
Giakis et al (1993)	Flx/Bup	11	13	50% reduction HAMD	27.2	0	4 (Flx)	2–33
Nair et al (1995)	Nor/Moc	38	36	HAM-D<10	31.6	22.2	11 (Nor)	3–∞
Schone and Ludwig (1993)	Par/Flx	54	52	50% reduction HAMD	37.0	16.0	5 (Par)	3–22
Hoyberg et al (1996)	Mir/Ami	56	59	CGI very much or much improvement	74.0	81.0	14 (Ami)	5–∞
Kyle et al (1996)	Cit/Ami	179	186	Marked reduction of MADRS	53.6	53.2	500 (Cit)	10–∞
Karlsson et al (2002)	Cit/Mia	140	149	MADRS<12	43.0	35.0	12 (Cit)	5–∞
Karlsson et al (2002)	Cit/Mia	140	149	50% reduction MADRS	33.6	26.8	15 (Cit)	6–∞
Smeraldi et al (1997)	Ven/Clo	55	58	CGI improved	74.0	69.0	20 (Ven)	5–∞

Table 4 *continued*

Authors	Drugs	N (drug 1)	N (drug 2)	Measure	Percentage response drug 1	Percentage response drug 2	NNT	95% CI
Mahapatra and Hackett (1997)	Ven/Doth	44	48	MADRS improvement	47.0	34.0	8 (Ven)	3–∞
Mahapatra and Hackett (1997)	Ven/Doth	44	48	HAM-D improvement	49.0	47.0	50 (Ven)	4–∞
Smeraldi et al (1997)	Ven/Trz	55	57	CGI improved	74.0	57.0	6 (Ven)	3–∞
Smeraldi et al (1997)	Clo/Trz	58	57	CGI improved	69.0	57.0	8 (Clo)	3–∞
Merideth et al (1984)	Nom/Imi	19	14	CGI improved	78.9	64.3	7 (Nom)	2–∞
Cohn et al (1984)	Nom/Imi	21	21	CGI improvement	82.0	82.0	∞	4–∞
Wakelin (1986)	Flv/Imi	33	29	CGI improved	79.0	65.0	7 (Flv)	3–∞
Hutchinson et al (1991)	Ami/Par	32	58	50% reduction HAMD	14.0	24.0	10 (Par)	4–∞

Ami, amitriptyline; Bup, bupropion; CGI, clinical global impression; CI, confidence interval; Cit, citalopram; CLO, clomipramine; Doth, dothiepin; Flv, fluvoxamine; Flx, fluoxetine; HAMD, Hamilton Depression Rating Scale; MADRS, Montgomery Asberg Depression Rating Scale; Mia, mianserin; Mir, mirtazapine; Moc, moclobemide; N, number; NNT, number needed to treat; Nor, nortriptyline; Par, paroxetine; Ser, sertraline; Trz, trazodone; Ven, venlafaxine.

Table 5 Adverse outcomes – numbers needed to harm (NNH).

Authors	Drugs	N (drug 1)	N (drug 2)	Measure	Percentage adverse drug 1	Percentage adverse drug 2	NNH	95% CI
Nair et al (1995)	Nor/Pla	38	36	Premature cessation of treatment	47.4	42.9	22 (Nor)	4–∞
Nyth et al (1992)	Cit/Pla	60	33	Side effects	37.0	25.0	8 (Cit)	3–∞
Nair et al (1995)	Moc/Pla	36	35	Premature cessation of treatment	58.3	42.9	6 (Moc)	3–∞
Tollefson et al (1995)	Flx/Pla	335	336	Early discontinuation	11.6	8.6	33 (Flx)	13–∞
Merideth et al (1984)	Imi/Pla	14	15	Premature cessation	57.1	60.0	34 (Pla)	3–∞
Merideth et al (1984)	Nom/Pla	19	15	Premature cessation	21.1	60.0	3 (Pla)	1–11
Merideth et al (1984)	Imi/Nom	14	19	Premature cessation	57.1	21.1	3 (Imi)	2–∞
Nair et al (1995)	Nor/Moc	38	36	Premature cessation	47.4	58.3	9 (Moc)	3–∞
Mahapatra and	Ven/Doth	44	48	Premature	7.0	8.0	100 (Doth)	8–∞

Table 5 *continued*

Authors	Drugs	N (drug 1)	N (drug 2)	Measure	Percentage adverse drug 1	Percentage adverse drug 2	NNH	95% CI
Hackett (1997)				cessation				
Hoyberg et al (1996)	Mirt/Ami	56	59	Premature cessation	26.0	19.0	14	5–∞
Cohn et al (1990)	Ser/Ami	161	80	Side effects	28.0	35.0	14 (Ami)	5–∞
Geretsegger et al (1994)	Par/Flx	54	52	Adverse effects	61.0	77.0	6 (Flx)	3–∞
Finkel and Richter (1995)	Ser/Nor	35	37	Discontinuation caused by side effects	12.8	24.3	9 (Nor)	3–∞
Kyle et al (1996)	Cit/Ami	179	186	Premature cessation of drug treatment	24.6	30.1	18 (Ami)	7–∞
Karlsson et al (2002)	Cit/Mia	140	149	Adverse reactions	84.3	87.9	28 (Mia)	9–∞
Smeraldi et al (1997)	Ven/Clo	55	58	Adverse effects	19.0	39.0	5 (Clo)	3–28
Smeraldi et al (1997)	Ven/Trz	55	57	Adverse effects	19.0	43.0	4 (Trz)	2–13
Smeraldi et al (1997)	Clo/Trz	58	57	Adverse effects	39.0	43.0	25 (Trz)	5–∞
Hutchinson et al (1991)	Ami/Par	32	58	Adverse events	63.0	34.0	3 (Ami)	2–15

Ami, amitriptyline; Bup, bupropion; CI, confidence interval; Cit, citalopram; Clo, clomipramine; Doth, dothiepin; Flv, fluvoxamine; Flx, fluoxetine; Mia, mianserin; Mir, mirtazapine; Moc, moclobemide; N, number; Nor, nortriptyline; Par, paroxetine; Pla, placebo; Ser, sertraline; Trz, trazodone; Ven, venlafaxine.

When the difference between the two treatments is not statistically significant, confidence intervals can be difficult to describe as they cross over zero. If the true absolute risk reduction (ARR) is zero, the NNT is infinite. Similarly, if the 95% confidence interval of the ARR crosses zero, then the corresponding limit of its 95% confidence interval is infinite.

Our analysis suggests that the majority of antidepressants evaluated by placebo-controlled trials in older people are effective, with relatively small NNTs, similar to those reported in younger patients. For fluoxetine, however, the analysis indicates a relatively high NNT and for moclobemide the confidence intervals include infinity. This therefore casts doubt on the efficacy of moclobemide and, to some degree, of fluoxetine in the treatment of depression in older people.

Only one of the head-to-head efficacy comparisons between antidepressants showed significant differences in NNT, paroxetine being significantly more likely than fluoxetine to lead to a 50% reduction in the score on the Hamilton Scale at 6 weeks. The confidence intervals are extremely wide for many trials, suggesting inadequate sample size. The data do, however, suggest true equivalence in efficacy for citalopram and amitriptyline. There is otherwise a consistent trend favouring SSRIs.

With the exception of nomifensine (which has now been discontinued) and imipramine, all antidepressants appear to produce more adverse effects than placebo, although in most cases the differences are not significant, with NNT 95% confidence intervals including infinity. The adverse effect data suggest only modest (but, again, consistent) superiority of SSRIs over TCAs. This is statistically significant in the comparison between paroxetine and amitriptyline. Venlafaxine has significantly fewer adverse effects than either clomipramine or trazodone.

Our analysis therefore supports the preferential use of SSRIs (with the possible exception of fluoxetine) and of venlafaxine in the treatment of depression in older people.

Ancillary medication

It is sometimes necessary for symptoms of depression such as sleep disturbance and anxiety to be treated before the antidepressant medication has begun to take effect. The former may be treated with hypnotics such as benzodiazepines, zopiclone or zolpidem (although relatively sedating antidepressants may also be tried), the latter by benzodiazepines or low-dose neuroleptics. Important principles to consider are avoiding polypharmacy as far as possible and limiting the period of co-administration by progressive reduction of the ancillary medication with a view to discontinuation as an antidepressant response (which should include improvement in sleep or anxiety symptoms) emerges.

Prevention of relapse and recurrence

Most relapses of depressive illness occur within the first year of an episode, and older patients may be at high risk of relapse for up to 2 years.

There have been relatively few studies of longer-term treatment following good initial response. In people with other previous episodes of depression, continued antidepressant treatment has been shown to be effective in preventing relapse for at least 2–3 years. The relative rate of risk of relapse over 2 years was two and a half times greater in a placebo group than in patients receiving the TCA dothiepin at 75 mg/day. Similar long-term efficacy in patients at high risk of relapse has been shown for nortriptyline in a trial lasting 3 years. Most other published trials have lacked placebo control, and there is insufficient RCT evidence for the efficacy of the newer agents, such as SSRIs, in the long-term treatment of depression overall. The exception is citalopram 20–40 mg which in a placebo controlled trial in responders at 8 weeks reduced the rates of recurrence from 68% to 32% over a 48 week period. None of the patients on 20 mg citalopram experienced a recurrence, (Klysner et al, 2002). There is, however, consistent open trial evidence that TCAs and SSRIs have similar prophylactic effects.

Psychological therapies, such as cognitive–behavioural therapy (CBT) and supportive psychotherapy may also reduce relapse rate, with the most powerful prophylactic effect reported resulting from combined antidepressant and interpersonal therapy (IPT).

Lithium is also widely used, either on its own or to augment an antidepressant, although the risk of adverse effects is high and specific precautions (discussed in Chapter 5) need to be taken before initiating lithium treatment. In particular, lithium carries a high risk of neurotoxicity in old age, particularly in the context of co-morbid dementia and/or Parkinson's disease.

In general antidepressants should, where possible, be continued (without any dose reduction) for at least 6 months after clinical recovery. Opportunistic monitoring of depressive symptoms should form part of any subsequent clinical contact. Treatment should be continued for at least 2 years (and perhaps indefinitely) in patients at high risk of relapse. Indicators of such high risk include a particularly severe index episode, two or more episodes in the previous 2 years, chronic physical illness or significant social stressors.

Refractory depression in old age

Depression in old age frequently fails to respond to initial treatment. The strategy below outlines a systematic way of dealing with this.

Patients with apparent treatment resistance should be fully re-evaluated (*Box 11*), with consideration of whether the original diagnosis was correct, previous treatment adequate (dosage and duration) and

---

Box 11   Refractory depression in old age.

Review	*Main options*
Adequacy of treatment:	ECT
dosage	Augmentation strategies
duration	Novel pharmacotherapies
compliance	
Appropriateness of treatment	
Maintenance factors	

adherence satisfactory. Possible physical (e.g. hypothyroidism, poorly controlled pain) or psychosocial (e.g. isolation, poor marital relationship) maintenance factors should also be considered.

If the above two strategies are used, the rate of non-response falls to 20%. Various pharmacological approaches to such 'true' refractory depression in older people have been evaluated. Within these, lithium augmentation has the strongest evidence base. Older patients who have failed to respond to treatment, and in whom other factors have been adequately addressed should be considered for adjuvant therapy. However, lower doses are required and the 'therapeutic window' for blood levels needs to be adjusted downwards to a range of about 0.4–0.9 mmol/l, with low levels in this range usually being better tolerated, particularly to avoid toxic responses resulting from age-related pharmacodynamic changes.

Other strategies include switching class of antidepressant, using combinations of antidepressants (such as TCA + SSRI) or using less 'mainstream' drugs such as methylphenidate or selegiline.

Antidepressants may be less effective in patients with psychotic depression. The combination of antidepressant and anti-psychotic may be effective in psychotic depression, although most of the evidence in support of this strategy comes from studies in younger people.

Antidepressants: switching and stopping

All antidepressants have the potential to cause withdrawal symptoms (*Box 12*). When they have been prescribed for 6 weeks or longer, they should not be stopped suddenly unless there is a side effect that makes this necessary. They should be withdrawn slowly, preferably over at least 4 weeks, with weekly decreases in dosage. The exception to this is fluoxetine which has a long half-life and active metabolites, and may be stopped abruptly. Usually, when switching antidepressants one drug should be reduced slowly, whereas the other is introduced with caution and the patient monitored for side effects. This is unnecessary when switching from one SSRI to another – however, there are few good reasons for such a switch.

Box 12   Antidepressant discontinuation syndrome.

- Dizziness
- Anxiety and agitation insomnia
- Flu-like symptoms
- Diarrhoea and abdominal spasm
- Paraesthesia
- Mood swings
- Nausea

Paroxetine has been particularly associated with withdrawal phenomena, especially dizziness and anxiety. One strategy that has been considered for those who have a severe withdrawal is switching to fluoxetine and then withdrawing it.

Potential dangers of simultaneously administering two antidepressants include serotonin syndrome (*Box 13*) and elevation of TCA levels by some SSRIs.

Box 13   Serotonin syndrome symptoms.

- Restlessness
- Tremor
- Shivering
- Myoclonus
- Confusion
- Convulsions
- Death

MAOIs have particular dangers in co-administration with other antidepressants, because the increase in peripheral tyramine can cause malignant hypertension. MAOIs should be withdrawn 2 weeks before giving other antidepressants. Equally, most other antidepressants should be withdrawn 2 weeks before giving MAOIs. The exception to this is fluoxetine which, because of its long half-life and active metabolites, should be withdrawn 5 or 6 weeks before giving MAOIs.

Other treatments

Electroconvulsive therapy

Although this book is about drug treatments in old age psychiatry, this chapter would not be complete without a brief mention of electrocon- vulsive therapy (ECT) and psychotherapy. ECT remains an important treatment option in very severe or treatment-resistant depression in old age. A meta-analysis of published studies revealed a 62% recovery and 21% substantial improvement. It is indicated particularly where depres- sive delusions are present, where retardation is marked, in patients whose fluid intake (secondary to loss of appetite and self-neglect) is poor enough to threaten renal function, and where suicide risk is considered high. Good anaesthetic support is essential. ECT may have to be delayed in very frail patients until their physical condition improves. ECT may be life-saving, particularly in the context of dehydration or suicidality. Its safety profile in older patients with depression is surprisingly good. A wide spectrum of clinical response, including anxiety symptoms, has been demonstrated. Unilateral electrode placement appears to be as effective as bilateral placement in older patients, but there is clearer evidence that unilateral electrode placement is associated with fewer memory-related side effects in this age group.

Psychological treatments

Psychological treatments are also underused in old age. This is partly because their availability is often limited. There is also a misconception that older people lack the psychological flexibility to benefit from psy- chotherapeutic interventions. Older people appear to respond particu- larly well to cognitive therapy for depression; this is effective both in an individual setting and (more economically) in groups. The focus is often on real or threatened losses (bereavement, physical health, financial security) and on fears of impending death. Interpersonal psychotherapy, which is widely used in the USA and increasingly so in Europe, has been shown to be effective in acute, continuation and maintenance treatment of depression in older people.

chapter 3

Co-morbid depression: depression in the context of other illnesses

Many studies have shown that older people with significant physical illness are considerably more likely to have important depressive symptoms than those fortunate enough to be physically healthy. Given the very high prevalence of physical ill health in older people (particularly very old people), this association, although no stronger than is found in younger people, is an important one. A further reason for being mindful of physical illness when an older person presents with depressive symptoms is that the co-morbid physical illness may be an important consideration in formulating a management plan. There is also evidence that depression may worsen the prognosis of coexistent physical illness and, equally, that depression may itself be more treatment resistant in the presence of significant physical morbidity.

There are several reasons why there should be such an association between physical illness and depression in old age (*Box 14*). Both conditions may be common and therefore coexist by coincidence. Physical illness may lead to appropriate depressive symptoms or a reactive depression. By the same token, depression (particularly if complicated by self-neglect and psychomotor retardation) may have adverse effects on physical health. Depression may also alter the wish to recover physically and, in particular, reduce adherence to treatments for co-morbid physical illness. The 5-item Geriatric Depression Scale (*Box 15*) has been developed to screen for depression in people with physical illness and has good psychometric properties. It has since been validated in Chilean

Box 14   Possible reasons for the association between physical illness and depression in old age.

- Coincidence
- Appropriate reaction
- Physical deterioration mediated by neglect
- Poor adherence to physical management
- Hypothalamic–pituitary–adrenal axis dysregulation

community dwelling patients, and geriatric outpatients in the USA. Depression is often associated with abnormalities of the hypothalamic–pituitary– adrenal axis; the resultant hypercortisolaemia may have adverse physical effects.

Where depressive symptoms are minor, understandable and transient, supportive care in the context of appropriate management of the physical illness may be sufficient. In many cases, however, symptoms are persistent and/or disabling. In such cases, appropriate, specific treatment of the depression may make a considerable difference to overall outcome. General practitioners, physicians and surgeons working with physically ill older people therefore need to be aware of the different ways that depression can present in the context of physical illness, how to distinguish between minor depressive symptoms and a full-blown depressive illness in physically ill patients, and how such depression can most safely and effectively be treated.

Despite its importance, the rate of detection of depression by hospital physicians is low – with many studies reporting that only 10–20% of cases in the general hospital setting are detected and still fewer treated. This probably reflects widespread ignorance of the relevant diagnostic criteria and aetiological factors and, more particularly, of how the presentation of depression can alter in the presence of poor physical health. Screening (which may be very effective in identifying depression 'cases' – *Box 15*) is seldom used. There may also be excessive reluctance to use potentially dangerous treatments.

Box 15   The 5-item Geriatric Depression Scale for use in people
with comorbid physical illness (From Hoyl et al, 1999)

1. Are you basically satisfied with your life? Y/<u>N</u>
2. Do you often get bored? <u>Y</u>/N
3. Do you often feel helpless? <u>Y</u>/N
4. Do you prefer staying at home rather than going out and doing new
   things? <u>Y</u>/N
5. Do you feel pretty worthless the way you are now? <u>Y</u>/N

Underlined answers score 1 point. Scores of ≥2 indicate probable depression.

Prevalence, clinical presentation and prognosis

Depressive symptoms occur in as many as 50% of older people on
general hospital wards, although reported rates depend crucially on age,
sex, type of ward and threshold for identifying depressive 'caseness'.
Community studies also find that older people with multiple physical
conditions have rates of depression that are much higher than in those
who are relatively fit. Some physical symptoms, including headache and
shortness of breath, have been found to be particularly strongly associated with depression, as have some specific diseases: stroke, Parkinson's
disease and malignant disease of which the patient is aware. Close monitoring and supportive management may be appropriate if the depressive
symptoms are mild and of short duration.

Depression often presents covertly in medically ill older people. Psy-
chosomatic presentations or apparent hypochondria may be very difficult to distinguish from 'true' symptoms of the coexisting physical
illness or illnesses. Disturbed sleep, pain, loss of appetite or weight,
fatigue, anxiety and thoughts of death are all common in physically ill
older people and may be 'driven' both by depression and by physical
morbidity. Not surprisingly, somatic symptoms are not very helpful in
identifying true depressive illness, although when their nature and

severity are difficult to explain in terms of the underlying physical pathology, depression should be considered.

Some clinical features are more specifically suggestive of depression that requires specific treatment in the presence of significant physical illness (*Box 16*). These include loss of interest and pleasure, a feeling that the illness is a punishment or of being a failure, suicidal thoughts or gestures, dissatisfaction with treatment, indecisiveness and prominent tearfulness. As well as these psychological and cognitive symptoms of depression, there are often somatizing symptoms, including disproportionate complaints of pain, the need for increased analgesics and hypnotics with little effect, and unexpectedly poor response to specific treatment of the physical illness. Background factors indicating increased vulnerability include a past psychiatric history (particularly of depression), significant cognitive impairment, relatively severe medical illness or (in surgical patients) postoperative complications.

Depressive symptoms are less likely to resolve in the presence of physical illness – although depression after stroke may be an exception. Both acute new physical illness and chronic health problems have been found to predict the persistence or recurrence of depression. In one study of older patients admitted to psychiatric care with depression, almost all those who were free of active physical pathology recovered fully,

---

Box 16   Pointers to depression in physically ill older people.

- Loss of interest
- Anhedonia
- Feeling punished
- Feeling a failure
- Suicidality
- Dissatisfaction
- Indecisiveness
- Tearfulness
- Increased complaints of pain
- Co-prescription of analgesics and hypnotics
- Lack of response to treatment

whereas most of those whose depression failed to respond to treatment had one or more physical illnesses at the time of initial admission.

Co-morbid depression in physically ill older people is linked to higher than expected chronicity and disability from physical illness, increased use of healthcare resources (particularly bed occupancy) and, most important of all, increased mortality from natural causes. The link between depression and mortality is particularly marked in the context of cardiac disease. It has been shown that depression is one of the most powerful predictors of cardiac mortality and sudden death in the year after acute myocardial infarction, even after allowing for other known clinical predictors of disease severity. Depression in older stroke victims and in people who fracture their hips is also associated with significantly higher mortality. In the latter group, the combination of depression and cognitive impairment is a particularly predictor of early death. Similar findings have been reported in patients followed up after acute hospitalization for a range of life-threatening illnesses. Although the group who were depressed did not have more severe physical illnesses, they did have a significantly poorer outcome over the next 28 days, with 47% (compared with only 10% of the non-depressed group) dying or having a serious complication.

Depression in dementia

Why is treating depression in dementia different from treating depression in patients without dementia?

Box 17 summarizes the differences in depression in people with compared with those without dementia. Depression in dementia may result from anatomical and biochemical changes in the brain, which are different to the changes occurring when a patient does not have dementia. Thus, the presentation and response to treatment may differ from depression in people without dementia. Dementia may, for example, alter the presentation of depression so that behavioural symptoms such as disruptive vocalization may be more prominent than cognitive symptoms such as guilt and worthlessness. As patients are unlikely to

---

Box 17   Why depression in dementia is different.

- Depression in dementia may result from anatomical changes in the brain
- Presentation of depression may be different with more prominent disruptive behaviour
- Depression in dementia may be more difficult to detect
- There are more practical difficulties in physical and psychological treatment if the patient has memory problems
- Depression in dementia has been shown to accelerate functional decline

---

remember their dominant mood and whether, for example, they have sleep difficulties or loss of appetite, depression in dementia may be more difficult to detect. In addition to the diagnostic difficulty, there may be practical obstacles in physical and psychological treatment, because the patient may forget to take tablets or may not be able to remember the contents of a therapeutic session. Depression in dementia is, however, important because not only does it lead to decreased quality of life but it also has been shown to accelerate functional decline.

Epidemiology of depression in dementia

There are huge variations in prevalence rates of depression, which have been reported with, for example, rates in clinic samples ranging from 6% to 38%. This may be because clinics have unrepresentative samples of people attending clinics for a variety of reasons and with different forms of dementias. A prevalence of moderate-to-severe depressive disorder, in patients with Alzheimer's disease (AD), of 20%, has been calculated, higher than in aged-matched community residents. The literature has consistently reported that depression is more common in vascular as opposed to Alzheimer's disease-type dementia. A recent study reported the rates of depression in a community sample of people with Alzheimer's disease (AD) and vascular dementia to be 3.2% and 21.2%, respectively. Depression is also found to be particularly common in dementia with Lewy bodies (DLB), with 38% of people with DLB being depressed in comparison to 15% of people with AD. Despite this, the persistence of depression in both diseases has been shown to be similar.

The effect of depression in dementia on caregivers

Caregivers of people with dementia are at increased risk of depression. The increased distress is particularly related to neuropsychiatric symptoms of dementia rather than cognitive symptoms (*Figure 2*). Caregiver morbidity has also been specifically linked to depression and demanding behaviour in the person with dementia, both of which are independent predictors for the caregiver. This caregiver depression often leads to the breakdown of care and the institutionalization of the person with dementia.

Measurement of depression in dementia

Depression in dementia can be difficult to diagnose, both because patients can forget their symptoms as discussed above and because there is an overlap of symptoms, e.g. lack of interest, between dementia and depression.

There are specialized scales that have been developed for the detection of depression in dementia; these work by formalizing the usual clinical approach of asking the carer about symptoms. The Cornell Scale for Depression in Dementia takes a different approach by synthesizing questions derived from an informant and by observation. Its 19 items cover anxiety, sadness, lack of reactivity to pleasant events, irritability, agitation, retardation, multiple physical complaints, loss of interest, appetite

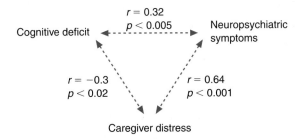

Figure 2 *Alzheimer's disease symptoms and caregiver distress.*

loss, weight loss, lack of energy, diurnal variation, difficulty falling asleep, multiple awakenings during sleep, early morning wakening, suicidal wishes or intent, self-depreciation, pessimism and mood-congruent delusions. Each item is rated on a 3-point scale. There may be several iterations as the rater seeks concordance between the caregiver's description and the observations of the patient, so that, although the internal validity and reliability are good, it takes between 20 and 30 minutes to administer.

Another approach is to use a scale that has been developed to measure neuropsychiatric symptoms, and which asks an informant about the frequency and severity of a range of non-cognitive symptoms of dementia, any of which can be caused by depression (see, for example, the Neuropsychiatric Inventory – see *Box 18*).

The evidence base for treating depression in dementia
Antidepressants for depression in dementia

If treatment is indicated because of the intensity or duration of symptoms, several drugs having been reported as being superior to placebo for depression in dementia. Citalopram has been found to improve not only depressed mood and panic symptoms but also recent memory, orientation and an inability to increase pace. There was a trend for patients prescribed moclobemide, in dosages of between 100 mg and 400 mg, to improve more than those on placebo. Sertraline had no advantage over placebo in a small study of nursing home residents, although both groups tended to improve over time. One study of nortriptyline versus placebo in nursing home residents found efficacy only in patients who

Box 18   Neuropsychiatric Inventory (NPI).

- Delusions
- Disinhibition
- Apathy/indifference
- Hallucinations
- Anxiety

- Elation/euphoria
- Irritability/lability
- Aberrant motor symptoms
- Dysphoria/depression
- Agitation/aggression

were not depressed. A study of clomipramine 25–100 mg in patients with dementia and depression or dysthymia found that, although clomipramine had superior efficacy as measured by the response of depressive symptoms, it had a mild adverse effect on cognition.

There have been some head-to-head trials of antidepressants in this field. In the first two, groups of patients responded well on depression scales to citalopram 20–40 mg/day and mianserin 30–60 mg/day for 12 weeks. Fatigue and somnolence were more common with mianserin and insomnia with citalopram. In the second, the effect of 20–40 mg paroxetine was compared with 50–100 mg imipramine. There was a significantly greater improvement in the patients taking paroxetine on the Cornell Scale, but a similar improvement using a general scale for depression. A third study compared 10 mg fluoxetine with 25 mg amitriptyline and found a high drop-out rate, particularly with amitriptyline, and no significant differences in response, although there was a tendency for patients on fluoxetine to do better.

Cholinesterase inhibitors for depression in dementia
The cholinesterase inhibitors have been reported to improve neuropsychiatric and depressive symptoms in people with AD. Most of the studies have been open label, but have consistently found rivastigmine, donepezil and galantamine to be associated with improvements in such symptoms as depressed mood, anxiety, irritability and aberrant motor activity.

Conclusions about treatment of depression in dementia
Symptoms tend to improve over time, although patients who have persistent and significant symptoms may respond to drug treatment. At present the most consistent and best results in this field are for paroxetine and citalopram.

Management of depression in people with other physical illnesses

The principles of management of depression in older people with co-morbid physical illness are essentially the same as for depression in general. The possibility of contraindications, adverse interactions with other drug treatment and side effects being more significant and disabling must be borne in mind. The danger of such side effects is, however, easy to exaggerate and must be offset against the greater danger of therapeutic nihilism.

Undertaking controlled trials of antidepressant treatments in elderly people presents formidable problems. Despite this, some (relatively small) trials have been successfully completed, and these provide some guidance towards clinical management decisions.

One study compared mianserin and maprotiline in 48 elderly physically ill individuals with major depression or dysthymia; 35 completed the trial. Overall improvement rates were only around 40%, although mianserin was significantly superior in terms of depression rating scores. Another study compared lofepramine (at a dose of 70 mg daily, lower than the usual therapeutic dose of 140 mg) with placebo in 63 depressed elderly medical in-patients; 46 patients completed the trial. Overall, improvement was similar in the two groups, but lofepramine was superior to placebo only in those with more severe depression. In contrast, placebo was associated with a significantly better outcome in the group with milder depression.

Evans et al (1997) carried out the largest placebo-controlled trial to date, in older medical patients with depression. Their active drug was the SSRI fluoxetine. The outcome in this study was that the difference in response rates (64% with fluoxetine, 38% with placebo) just failed to reach statistical significance. *Post-hoc* analyses showed fluoxetine to be significantly superior in those who completed 5 weeks of treatment and in those with more severe physical illnesses.

Another trial of fluoxetine compared it with the tricyclic antidepressant (TCA) nortriptyline in 64 hospitalized patients who had severe depression and heart disease; the mean age of the patients was 70. Response to nortriptyline was significantly better than that to fluoxetine (67% vs 23%). This trial was not, however, randomized or masked.

The psychostimulant methylphenidate is widely used in the USA in the treatment of frail older medical patients with depression who have 'turned their faces to the wall'. A small placebo-controlled crossover study of methylphenidate against placebo showed the drug to be well tolerated with minimal cardiovascular effects. A rapid improvement in mood was seen in several patients and the difference against placebo reached statistical significance. It is, however, unclear whether this was simply a stimulant effect rather than an effect on the 'core' depressive symptoms.

Despite the relatively high risk of toxicity that it carries in frail elderly people, lithium augmentation has been specifically reported to be beneficial in physically ill elderly patients with refractory depression.

In the clinical situation, it is important to be alert to contraindications to antidepressants, the co-administration of drugs for physical illness with which they might interact adversely and the emergence of disabling side effects. The danger of toxic effects in overdose may also be greater in patients with physical co-morbidity. The danger of focusing on such potential problems is, however, that it is easy to exaggerate the risks and to forget the benefits, and therapeutic nihilism is a particular trap in elderly medical patients with co-existing depression.

Practical considerations for specific medical co-morbidities

Cardiovascular disease

Older people are at high risk of both ischaemic heart disease and heart failure. Dysrythmias (particularly atrial fibrillation and heart block) are also common.

In general, SSRIs are preferable to TCAs (which increase heart rate, prolong the Q–T_c interval and affect cardiac contractility), although fluvoxamine and citalopram may also be cardiotoxic in overdose.

Controlled trial data in patients with cardiovascular disease (not specific to older people) suggest that paroxetine is safer than nortriptyline, and that citalopram also seldom exacerbates existing cardiac morbidity. Nefazodone may be considered if a sedative effect is required. Moclobemide is also virtually free of cardiac side effects.

In patients who have had a recent myocardial infarction, antidepressants should be avoided for at least 2 months if possible. Sertraline is the only antidepressant to have been studied extensively in patients post-myocardial infarction, and appears to be effective and relatively safe. Most newer antidepressants are safe in patients with angina, but trazodone and nefazodone (as well as the TCAs) should probably be avoided.

Depressed patients with heart failure should avoid antidepressants that cause postural hypotension – these include the TCAs, nefazodone, trazodone and venlafaxine. These drugs may also augment the effect of anti-hypertensives. Hypertension may, however, also be exacerbated by venlafaxine. Some anti-hypertensives (methyldopa, lipid-soluble β blockers such as propranolol) may trigger or worsen depression, and alternative anti-hypertensive treatment should be considered in patients who become depressed. SSRIs (particularly citalopram and with the possible exception of fluvoxamine) are relatively safe in patients with arrhythmias. Antidepressants may interact adversely with warfarin, which is increasingly being used in older patients with atrial fibrillation or stroke. Several antidepressants may alter the anticoagulant effects of warfarin which needs to be monitored carefully. This is a result of their extensive protein binding which may displace warfarin (TCAs, SSRIs except citalopram, trazodone, nefazodone) and their complex actions as substrates for, or inhibitors of, the cytochrome P450 isoenzymes that control warfarin metabolism (SSRIs, trazodone, nefazodone, venlafaxine, moclobemide, monoamine oxidase inhibitors [MAOIs], TCAs). Citalopram is probably least likely to alter the international normalized ratio (INR) in patients receiving warfarin.

Renal failure

Mild renal failure is very common in old age. It must be remembered that, as a result of age-related loss of muscle bulk, serum creatinine levels may be misleadingly low. TCAs have active metabolites that are excreted by the kidney. In patients with renal failure, TCAs should therefore be given in divided doses and tolerability monitored closely. Plasma level monitoring (where available) may also be useful. Lofepramine is excreted largely unchanged through the kidney and is best avoided in patients with severe renal failure. Among the SSRIs, citalopram can be given to patients with mild or moderate renal failure in normal doses. Fluxoetine should be given at lower than normal doses (10 mg/day or 20 mg on alternate days); paroxetine is also best given at 10 mg/day. There are limited data available on the use of sertraline or fluvoxamine. No dosage adjustment is necessary for moclobemide. Venlafaxine clearance is considerably reduced in renal failure; the dose should be reduced by 50% in mild or moderate renal failure and the drug avoided in severe renal failure.

Liver failure

In view of their extensive hepatic metabolism, most antidepressants should be given in reduced doses to patients with hepatic failure. Probably the safest antidepressants to use are the TCA imipramine and the SSRIs paroxetine or citalopram. The (already very long) half-life of fluoxetine and its major metabolite norfluoxetine are increased by about 50% and doses (or their frequency) should be halved. Doses of moclobemide and venlafaxine should also be reduced by at least half. Fluvoxamine and nefazodone have been noted occasionally to impair liver function. Several drugs are contraindicated in patients with liver failure, including lofepramine, sertraline, amitriptyline and dothiepin.

Parkinson's disease

Parkinson's disease (PD) is a common condition in older people; depression is found in up to 50% of PD patients. Treatment of depression in PD patients is thus often required. TCAs are effective and their anticholinergic effects may actually improve the extrapyramidal symptoms at the core of PD. They may, however, reduce absorption of levodopa and therefore worsen PD symptoms. Imipramine, nortriptyline and lofepramine have been most extensively evaluated. SSRIs have also been used, although they may cause tremor. Some SSRIs (paroxetine, fluoxetine) have been reported to worsen the range of motor symptoms in PD patients. MAOIs (including moclobemide) may trigger hypertensive crises in patients on levodopa and may also interact adversely with selegiline (itself a MAO-B inhibitor). Selegiline may itself have some antidepressant efficacy, especially at high doses (60 mg/day), in which context it is no longer MAO-B selective and requires tyramine restriction.

Epilepsy

Patients who develop depressive symptoms post-ictally usually do not require antidepressants; the main pharmacological strategy is to modify anti-epileptic drug treatment to reduce the frequency and severity of the seizures. Depression does, however, often occur unrelated to seizures in people with epilepsy and may be associated with particularly high risk of suicide. Some anti-epileptic drugs may exacerbate depression and should be avoided, including vigabatrin, primidone and phenobarbital (phenobarbitone). In contrast, others (carbamazepine, valproate) may have beneficial effects on depressed mood. Where antidepressants are required, the SSRIs (fluoxetine, sertraline) and moclobemide are relatively safe. Mianserin and clomipramine reduce seizure threshold significantly and are best avoided. Cognitive therapy and (paradoxically) electroconvulsive treatment (ECT) may also be effective.

Stroke

As depression frequently resolves spontaneously in stroke patients, antidepressant treatment should be restricted to those patients with severely persistent or disabling symptoms.

There have also been several controlled trials in the more specific context of stroke in (predominantly) older depressed patients. Nortriptyline has been found to be superior to placebo in the treatment of post-stroke depression. Only 14 of the 34 patients in the study were on active treatment: three developed antidepressant-related acute confusional states. There is a modest benefit for trazodone compared with placebo in reducing levels of dependency in stroke patients. Not all of those included were, however, clinically depressed at the outset and the primary outcome measure was dependency rather than depression. Another SSRI, citalopram, has been reported to be superior to placebo in post-stroke depression, although the spontaneous recovery rate was also high. The same group has reported citalopram to be effective in relieving the syndrome of persistent and abnormal tearfulness that is sometimes found after stroke.

The main practical considerations in choosing antidepressant therapy for stroke patients are the risk of worsening cognitive impairment, precipitating seizures and avoiding adverse interactions with other drugs such as warfarin. Aspirin is also often given following an ischaemic stroke; it may increase free plasma concentrations of highly protein-bound antidepressant drugs such as the TCAs, trazodone and most SSRIs. For these reasons and in view of the specific evidence base summarized above, citalopram may be the antidepressant of first choice for stroke patients.

Conclusions

The coexistence of depression and physical morbidity in old age worsens the prognosis of both. Evidence is growing that such depression can respond to active treatment, although possible adverse effects of antidepressants on the co-morbid physical illness must be considered carefully. Antidepressant treatment should always be seen as part of an overall management plan that addresses the specific physical problem(s) and resultant disability, as well as the social and psychological context. Close links between physician and psychiatrist are important to ensure that the possibility of significant co-morbid depression is considered in the initial assessment and subsequent care of elderly patients admitted to acute or chronic hospital beds.

Anxiety disorders

Several studies have examined the prevalence of different anxiety disorders in community-based populations (*Box 19*). The prevalence rates for phobias range from less than 1% to 11.7%; for generalized anxiety the range is between 1.4 and 7.3%. The variability in these findings probably reflects the use in some of specific case-finding instruments designed for elderly patients, e.g. the lower estimates suggest the need to have experienced the phobic reaction over the last month when many older people have completely avoided these stimuli. There is a general consensus that panic disorder is extremely rare in old age although panic attacks may occur comorbidly with other disorders.

Phobic disorders

Phobic disorders consist of persistent or recurrent irrational fear of an object, activity or situation that results in the compelling desire to avoid

---

Box 19   The range of anxiety disorders.

- Phobic disorders
- Generalized anxiety disorder
- Panic disorder
- Post-traumatic stress disorder

the phobic stimulus. This reduces the fear and is thus rewarding, so avoidance increases. In old age, the disorders are associated with higher rates of medical and other psychiatric morbidity, but are frequently found in the absence of other psychiatric disorders. Most specific phobias are early onset and continue into adult life. Most late-onset phobias are agoraphobia and are precipitated by traumatic experience or acute physical ill-health. Individuals with one phobia may develop another. Fear of crime is particularly common in old age, leading to fear of going out and night-time fearfulness. Social phobias in old age have usually developed earlier in life and persisted; they tend to be chronic and unremitting.

Co-morbidity with agoraphobia, specific phobia, depression and alcohol abuse is common. Elderly people rarely seek treatment and are often content to arrange their lives so that the phobic object is not part of it, e.g. never travel on the underground. Phobias do not, in general, seem to reduce life satisfaction. Cognitive–behavioural treatment is favoured over pharmacological interventions, although antidepressants may be useful in those with co-morbid depression (see Chapter 2). Anxiolytics provide only symptomatic relief and are best avoided because of their potential for dependency.

Generalized anxiety disorder

Generalized anxiety disorder consists of generalized, persistent anxiety, with motor tension, restlessness, tachycardia, tachypnoea, other autonomic symptoms, apprehensiveness and hypervigilance. It usually runs a chronic course. It is unusual to find it in older people without co-morbid depression. Coexistent medical conditions can complicate the situation. Patients are high service users, although they may not present complaining of anxiety or depression. If associated with depression, the depressive illness should be treated and most patients recover (see Chapter 2). Benzodiazepines have been the mainstay of treatment, but dependence and adverse effects should limit their use to very short-term management only.

Panic disorder

Panic disorder (which, as stated above, is rare in old age) is characterized by recurrent attacks of panic, with intense fear often of death accompanied by severe somatic anxiety symptoms. The patient often feels that he or she must escape from the situation. It usually runs a chronic course but may remit spontaneously or become less disabling secondary to reduced rates of social interaction in old age. It may, albeit rarely, occur anew in older people. Panic disorder with onset earlier in life is associated with depression, alcohol abuse, increased suicide risk and higher cardiovascular morbidity. Part of the explanation for the low prevalence in elderly people may be that sufferers may not survive into old age. Antidepressants are the pharmacological anti-panic agents of choice with selective serotonin reuptake inhibitors (SSRIs) increasingly used in preference to tricyclic antidepressants (see Chapter 2). Paroxetine and citalopram are licensed for this indication and the dose should gradually be increased to 40 mg if tolerated.

Benzodiazepines are efficacious for symptom control, but can only be used very short term because of undesirable side effects, such as memory loss, hangover, ataxia and dependence. Cognitive–behavioural therapy can be effective. The long-term outcome is improved by a combination drug and cognitive–behavioural approach.

Post-traumatic stress disorder

Post-traumatic stress disorder (PTSD) occurring earlier in life can be associated with disabilities persisting into old age. Traumatic events in old age can trigger similar PTSD reactions to those occurring in younger victims. The symptom profile is the same as with younger people who re-experience the trauma, hyperarousal and avoidance. Symptoms may be persistent or intermittent. The intensity of the physiological response to the original trauma may be the most significant predictor of a poor outcome. Further stressful life events can slow recovery, which may also be hindered by drug and alcohol abuse; these may themselves be triggered by PTSD.

PTSD can impair people's ability to deal with subsequent life stresses and symptoms may therefore resurface among older people who have had traumatic pasts, such as refugees, war victims and holocaust survivors. PTSD probably responds best to a combination of supportive therapeutic relationship, antidepressants and cognitive–behavioural therapy. There are no controlled trials in this age group.

chapter 5

Mania

Prevalence and classification

Community studies suggest a very low prevalence of mania in old age (< 1/1000) reflecting the high mortality of younger patients with bipolar illness, effective treatment with mood stabilizers (see below) and the tendency for mania to 'burn out' in long-term survivors of early onset mania. Mania is, however, relatively common in older hospital cohorts, representing 4–8% of psychiatric in-patient samples and as many as 12% of psychiatric admissions for mood disorders.

The Toronto group have suggested four main subgroupings of mania in older people (*Box 20*): primary bipolar disorder (recurrence in old age of early onset bipolar illness); latent bipolar disorder (first manic episode in late life after multiple depressive episodes, with the 'switch' possibly related to cerebrovascular disease); unipolar mania (early onset but no history of depressive episodes); and secondary mania, triggered (or

---

Box 20 Typology of mania in old age.

- Primary bipolar disorder
- Latent bipolar disorder
- Unipolar mania
- Secondary mania (disinhibition syndrome)

caused) by concurrent (usually cerebrovascular or cardiovascular) physical illness.

Clinical features

The clinical features of mania in older people are similar to those found in younger patients and are summarized in *Box 21*, which is based on the DSM-IV (*Diagnostic and Statistical Manual of Mental Disorders, 4th edn*) criteria. Behavioural disturbance (dramatic physical overactivity, violence, criminal behaviour, infectious euphoria and grandiosity) is usually less florid, however. Subjective confusion or perplexity is relatively prominent in older people with mania; true cognitive impairment is also commonly found. A 'mixed' picture, with features of depression as well as of mania, is also sometimes found in old age. Adverse life events, particularly episodes of illness, may be particularly important in precipitating manic episodes in older people.

First episode mania in very late life with no previous psychiatric history is usually associated with co-morbid neurological disorder, particularly with cerebrovascular disease. Such 'secondary mania' (which is also sometimes referred to in a neurological context as 'disinhibition syndrome') is almost invariably associated with some degree of cognitive impairment. Neuroimaging often reveals white matter hyperintensities

---

Box 21   Clinical features of mania.

- Elation
- Irritability
- Disinhibition
- Aggression
- Subjective confusion
- Pressure of speech
- Flight of ideas
- Grandiosity

and there is an overrepresentation of right-sided focal brain lesions, particularly in the orbitofrontal region. Family history and prior psychiatric disturbance are uncommon in secondary mania.

Prognosis of mania in older people

Two studies have followed cohorts of older bipolar patients for a mean of 6 years and compared their results with those for older people with unipolar depression. Mortality in mania is high (about 50% at 6 years compared with 20% in the depressed comparison groups) and mainly from associated cerebrovascular disease. The psychiatric prognosis in survivors is, however, surprisingly good with almost three-quarters symptom free and living independently.

Management of mania in old age

In view of the strong association between mania and physical (particularly cerebrovascular) co-morbidity, full physical evaluation is essential. Cerebrovascular risk factors such as hypertension and diabetes should be identified and treated. Neuroimaging should be seen as an important and perhaps essential part of the initial evaluation of a first episode mania.

The principles of drug treatment are similar to those in younger patients with mania. If the patient is on antidepressants, they should be withdrawn. Drug doses (particularly of lithium) will generally be smaller. There is, however, a dearth of controlled clinical trial data in older people and most randomized controlled trials (RCTs) have a cut-off age of 65 or less. Anti-psychotic drugs (particularly the atypicals – see Chapter 6) are widely used in acute symptomatic treatment. Current practice in all patients and, in particular, in older patients is, however, increasingly to use mood-stabilizing drugs as first-line treatment, because they appear to have powerful acute anti-manic effects and the dangers of polypharmacy are thereby minimized. Patients with 'rapid cycling' disorder may be particularly difficult to treat effectively; carbamazepine alone or in combination with lithium may be useful.

The range of drugs used is summarized in *Box 22*.

> Box 22   Physical treatments for bipolar disorder in older people.
>
> - Lithium
> - Valproate
> - Carbamazepine
> - Other anticonvulsants:
>   gabapentin
>   lamotrigine
>   topiramate
>   benzodiazepines
> - anti-psychotics (atypicals may have mood-stabilizing effects)
> - Other drugs: calcium channel blockers
> - Electroconvulsive treatment

First-line treatments

The dose range, probable mechanisms of action and most important side effects of the three most widely used mood stabilizers (lithium, sodium valproate and carbamazepine) are shown in *Table 6*.

Lithium

Lithium is widely used as a mood stabilizer and in potentiating partial or absent responses to antidepressants in refractory depression (see Chapter 2). Lithium also has a useful acute anti-manic effect. At the time of writing, no controlled clinical trials of lithium in older manic patients have been published.

Lithium has a wide range of pharmacological actions (see *Table 6* and see Chapter 7). It is taken up by cells more readily than it is extruded, and can substitute for other cations (calcium and magnesium as well as sodium and potassium). It inhibits both cyclic AMP and phosphoinositide second messenger system. Lithium enhances serotonin (5HT or 5-hydroxytryptamine) responsiveness and prevents the development of compensatory supersensitivity in response to receptor blockers.

Table 6 Drugs most commonly used to treat bipolar disorder in older people.

Drug	Dosage	Actions	Side effects	Comments
Lithium	Usually 200–600 mg/day Monitor to maintain therapeutic range 0.4–0.9 mmol/l. Aim for low end of range	Interaction with cationic systems Inhibition of second messengers Enhanced 5HT release Prevention of compensatory receptor supersensitivity	Neurotoxicity (25%) Fine tremor polyuria Parkinsonism Myxoedema Leukocytosis Diarrhoea Vomiting Psoriasis T-wave flattening Sick sinus syndrome Weight gain	Available as carbonate, citrate and in slow-release form Narrow therapeutic range Need baseline TFTs, U&Es, ECG Side effects lead to: reduced compliance must be distinguished from toxicity (Table 7)
Valproate	1000–1500 mg/day Aim at 50–90 mg/l	Enhanced GABA and 5HT activity Reduction in ACTH and cortisol levels	Vomiting Tremor Ataxia Weight gain Rash Confusion Flapping tremor	Momomeric and dimeric forms available May be combined with lithium (especially useful in rapid cycling patients)

Table 6 *continued*

Drug	Dosage	Actions	Side effects	Comments
Carbamazepine	Usually up to 800 mg/day in divided doses Keep serum level <9 mg/l	? Anti-kindling effect ? Potentiation of 5HT ? NMDA receptor blockade ? ↓ Ca^{2+} channel activation	Nausea Dizziness Ataxia Diplopia Nystagmus Headache Hyponatraemia Maculopapular rash (15%) Leukopenia Agranulocytosis Aplastic anaemia	Slow release formulation may reduce side effects Rashes, fever, sore throat may herald agranulocytosis Particularly useful in secondary mania

5HT, serotonin; GABA, γ-aminobutyric acid; NMDA, *N*-methyl-D-aspartate; TFTs, thyroid function tests; U&Es, urea and electrolytes

It is therefore not surprising that lithium causes a wide range of side effects (see *Table 6*). The most important of these are hypothyroidism (raised thyroid-stimulating hormone or TSH in about 25% of patients and clinical myxoedema in 10%); polyuria and polydipsia (secondary to inappropriate antidiuretic hormone [ADH] secretion), weight gain and fine tremor. Older people may develop more prominent neurological side effects including parkinsonism; those with pre-existing neurological disease (such as Parkinson's disease) or cognitive impairment are particularly vulnerable. Lithium can also cause ECG changes (T-wave flattening or inversion) and more rarely sinus node arrythmias. Leukocytosis is common but reversible and usually not clinically significant.

Lithium is excreted by the kidney and may accumulate rapidly if renal function is impaired or in the context of sodium depletion. Older people being started on lithium should have a baseline estimation of thyroid, renal and cardiac function. Even if their renal function is within the normal range, they usually require half the dose given to younger adults and are particularly vulnerable to lithium toxicity even at blood levels within the conventional adult 'therapeutic' range. Target blood levels for older patients should therefore be closely monitored and kept between 0.4 and 0.9 mmol/l, as far as possible at the lower end of the range. This is usually achieved with doses of between 200 and 600 mg/day. Initial dosage is 200 mg daily.

Angiotensin-converting enzyme (ACE) inhibitors, diuretics (especially thiazides) and non-steroidal anti-inflammatory drugs (with the exception of aspirin) may all enhance lithium toxicity by reducing its excretion by the kidney. The combination of verapamil and lithium may cause both neurotoxicity and bradycardia.

Lithium toxicity commonly occurs in older people for a variety of reasons, including erratic compliance, co-administered drugs and deteriorating renal function. It can rapidly become life threatening. Its clinical features (summarized in *Table 7*) are predominantly gastrointestinal and neurological; there is considerable overlap with the side effects seen at therapeutic blood levels. Gastrointestinal manifestations of mild lithium toxicity include nausea and diarrhoea. Vomiting is an indication of more serious toxicity. All these gastrointestinal symptoms also aggravate the toxicity by causing sodium depletion. Neurological manifestations may be further divided into motor and cognitive symptoms. Mild toxicity causes a more severe fine tremor than is usually seen at therapeutic levels and may also cause mild impairment of concentration. Signs of moderate toxicity include coarse tremor, ataxia, slurred speech, drowsiness and disorientation. Severe toxicity is indicated by more marked neurological disturbance which may include incontinence, choreiform movements, myoclonus, seizures, incontinence and (ultimately) coma.

Anticonvulsants

Anticonvulsants have long been used in the treatment of mood disorders. Their beneficial effects were first apparent in the form of improved mood in patients with epilepsy and co-morbid affective disorder. Their well-established efficacy in bipolar disorder in patients without epilepsy has led to the 'kindling' theory, which suggests that mood disorders might sensitize limbic areas much as drug-induced fits can, in animal models, trigger endogenous epilepsy.

Anticonvulsants vary widely in their pharmacological properties but many such drugs have similar actions in enhancing inhibitory neurotransmitters (particularly γ-aminobutyric acid [GABA]), reducing the

Table 7 Clinical features of lithium toxicity.

	Gastrointestinal	*Motor*	*Cognitive*
Mild	Nausea Diarrhoea	Fine tremor	Poor concentration
Moderate	Vomiting	Ataxia Slurred speech Coarse tremor	Drowsiness Disorientation
Severe		Incontinence Choreiform movements Myoclonus	Seizures Coma

activity of excitatory neurotransmitters and altering ion channels in nerve cell membranes.

Valproate

Valproate is available in monomeric (sodium valproate) and dimeric (semi-sodium valproate–divalproex) forms. It has a half-life of 8–20 hours and is metabolized mainly by oxidation. It is a weak inhibitor of cytochrome P450 2D6. Its main mechanism of action is thought to be facilitation of GABA neurotransmission; it may also act as a serotoninergic enhancer and reduce cortisol and ACTH levels.

Valproate is usually well tolerated by older people and appears to be very effective as an acute anti-manic agent (although perhaps slightly less effective than lithium) and mood stabilizer, although controlled trial evidence in older patients with mania is lacking. The usual dose range in older people is 1000–1500 mg/day (in divided doses), maintaining serum levels around 50–90 mg/l. Its main side effects (which often respond well to dose reduction) are gastrointestinal disturbances, sedation, ataxia and skin rashes.

Carbamazepine

Carbamazepine has a tricyclic structure. It is highly protein bound, has a short half-life (7 h) and is metabolized via cytochrome P450 1A2 and 3A4 isoenzymes. A wide range of drugs (including erythromycin, cimetidine, calcium channel blockers and fluoxetine) increase carbamazepine levels. Carbamazepine is also a cytochrome P450 enzyme inducer and thereby induces its own metabolism, as well as decreasing plasma levels of several drugs including haloperidol and warfarin.

Its mode of anti-manic and mood-stabilizing action is unclear, although anti-kindling effects, NMDA (*N*-methyl-D-aspartate) receptor blockade, central 5HT potentiation and reduced calcium channel activation may all be involved. As with valproate, there is a lack of controlled clinical trials with carbamazepine in older people. It may have a particular role (alone or in combination with lithium) in the treatment of rapid-cycling bipolar disorder.

Carbamazepine has a wide range of side effects. Older people are particularly vulnerable to neurotoxic effects, which can include dizziness, ataxia, headache and drowsiness. Nausea is also common. Hyponatraemia can occur through potentiation of ADH. An itchy maculopapular rash occurs in up to 15% of patients treated with carbamazepine. Subclinical leukopenia is common, particularly when treatment with carbamazepine is initiated; agranulocytosis and aplastic anaemia are rare but very serious side effects. Carbamazepine dosage for older people is usually initiated at 100 mg twice daily and maintained between 400 and 800 mg/day in divided doses, aiming to maintain plasma levels below 9 mg/l. Slow-release preparations not only allow simpler dosage regimens but may also reduce side effects.

Second-line treatments

Again there is little evidence of the most efficacious treatment to use. Usually patients at the beginning of an acute episode will take days or weeks on a mood stabilizer before it is effective. Although anti-psychotics can treat the symptoms, they may cause mood to decrease and precipitate a depressive episode. They also have numerous side effects (see Chapter 6). In the interim, sleep disturbance, overactivity and irritability may respond to a small dose of benzodiazepines. Short-acting ones should be used to decrease hangover effects, e.g. lorazepam 0.5–1 mg three times a day. The effects should be evaluated and the drug withdrawn as symptoms begin to resolve. If they do not, a third-line treatment should be used and the drug withdrawn because, if patients are left on benzodiazepine for more than a few weeks, they are likely to become dependent.

Third-line treatments

Anti-psychotics (see Chapter 6) remain in wide use for the treatment of acute mania. Dosages used are as for non-affective psychoses, although the aim is to achieve acute symptom control pending mood stabilization with lithium and/or an anticonvulsant.

Typical anti-psychotics carry a very significant side-effect burden and it must be remembered that both increasing age and affective disorder increase the risk of tardive dyskinesia. Atypical anti-psychotics are better tolerated and are increasingly being used in older patients with mania. It has been suggested that some atypical anti-psychotics, such as clozapine and olanzapine (which has recently been licensed for treatment of mania), may have mood-stabilizing properties.

Fourth-line treatments

A combination of mood stabilizers and newer anticonvulsants is widely used to treat younger patients with mania, although evidence for their efficacy in old age remains very limited. Lamotrigine blocks fast sodium channels and reduces excitatory neurotransmitter release. It appears to be well tolerated and may be beneficial in refractory bipolar disorder. Minor neurological side effects and rashes are common. Its long half-life (30 h) permits single daily dosing. It does not cause cognitive impairment which, together with its low (50%) protein binding and lack of effects on cytochrome P450 enzymes, make it a relatively safe drug for older people. Caution is required if it is combined with valproate or carbamazepine. Gabapentin is a recently introduced anticonvulsant that appears to have mood-stabilizing properties, as well as being useful in the treatment of neuropathic pain. Case studies suggest that it may be effective in resistant mania in old age, particularly in combination with lithium, valproate or carbamazepine. Like lamotrigine, its protein-bound fraction is low and it is free of significant interactions. Its plasma half-life is short. At doses of up to 2000 mg/day it is usually well tolerated, although mild neurological side effects (drowsiness, ataxia, tremor) are not uncommon.

Mood stabilizers and drug interactions

The most important drug interactions related to lithium use in elderly people cause neurotoxicity, particularly alterations in conscious level and tremor. ACE inhibitors, diuretics (especially thiazides) and non-steroidal anti-inflammatory drugs may all enhance lithium toxicity by reducing its excretion by the kidney. The combination of verapamil and lithium may cause both neurotoxicity and bradycardia.

Valproate is highly protein bound and is a weak inhibitor of cytochrome P450 2D6. Its half-life is significantly increased by co-administered cimetidine.

Carbamazepine-related interactions are also mainly metabolically induced. The selective serotonin reuptake inhibitors fluoxetine and flu-voxamine, the H_2-receptor antagonist cimetidine and the analgesic dex-tropropoxyphene may all cause carbamazepine toxicity by reducing its metabolism. The anticoagulant effect of warfarin may be reduced by co-administered carbamazepine.

chapter 6

Paranoid psychoses in older people

Psychotic symptoms can occur in older people in the context of all major mental illness and pharmacotherapy is a mainstay of treatment. This chapter concentrates on drug treatment for older people with paranoid illnesses that are not caused by a dementing illness, although older people with dementia and affective illnesses are also often treated with anti-psychotic drugs and the detailed information about these drugs is found in this chapter. Within the context of dementia, anti-psychotic drugs are often used for behavioural and psychiatric symptoms of dementia (BPSD), as well as for psychosis in dementia. The only published trials of anti-psychotic drugs that have been limited to older people have been in people with dementia. These are discussed in Chapter 7. As there are no trials that report the results in older people with paranoid illnesses, much of the information here is inferred from work in younger people.

The name of the illness

The onset of schizophrenia-like psychotic illness later in life, which is not the result of an organic or affective disorder, has been referred to as late-onset schizophrenia-like psychosis, paraphrenia, late paraphrenia and late-onset schizophrenia (*Box 23*). The international consensus statement published in 2000 refers to late-onset schizophrenia-like psychosis and very-late-onset schizophrenia-like psychosis, which occur

Box 23 Names for paranoid illnesses beginning in later life.

- Paraphrenia
- Late paraphrenia
- Late-onset schizophrenia
- Persistent delusional disorders
- Late life schizophrenia
- Late-onset schizophrenia-like psychosis
- Very late-onset schizophrenia-like psychosis

with onset in middle or old age. After a systematic review of the literature, those involved felt that these terms had face validity and clinical utility, and that general adoption of these terms would foster systematic investigation.

More circumscribed delusional disorders also occur in late life; these are referred to below as persistent delusional disorders. In addition, there are an increasing number of patients with long-standing psychotic illness (usually schizophrenia) who 'graduate' to old age.

The original concept of paraphrenia referred to the first onset of persecutory delusions and associated hallucinations after the age of 60 years, in the absence of an affective or organic psychosis. It may thus be viewed as schizophrenia or a schizophrenia-like illness in old age and is referred to as late life schizophrenia in *International Classification of Diseases*, 10th edn (ICD-10).

Who have late life paranoid illnesses?

It is unclear how common these paranoid illnesses are. Recent community studies have found that 2–4% of the older population had delusions or hallucinations over the past month, but that many of these symptoms were in the context of dementia. There is clearly a problem with epidemiological survey data because people who are suspicious, by the very nature of the condition, are far less likely than the rest of the population to cooperate with survey investigators. This probably results in considerable underestimation of the true community prevalence. There is relatively good consensus that late-onset schizophrenia is more common in women than in men (*Box 24*). Patients tend to be socially isolated. Their isolation is often chronic and may well be secondary to personality traits. They are predominantly unmarried women without close family or personal attachments. Those who do marry often end up divorced or separated. This social isolation creates an environment that allows the individual to become preoccupied in her own world. The social isolation can be further accentuated by sensory impairment. Patients often come to the attention of services because they complain to the police and neighbours with bizarre accusations over a period of time or because of neighbourly concern triggered by extreme self-neglect.

Box 24 Risk factors for late-life paranoid disorders.

- Female sex
- Social isolation
- Single, divorced or separated
- Sensory impairment

Mental state

On mental state assessment, there are no qualitative differences between the positive symptoms of early and those of late-onset schizophrenia. It may be difficult to elicit symptoms from patients who tend to be distrustful and hostile. Delusions are central. Organized delusional systems are common, with the frequency of paranoid and systematized delusions increasing in line with age. Sexual themes are common in women. Delusions of influence and passivity phenomena are frequently reported. Patients may describe their bodies as being controlled, or complain that some power affects them and they are made to do things against their will. Hallucinations are frequently experienced and are often in several modalities. Auditory hallucinations are the most common and usually have an accusatory and/or insulting content. Hallucinations of bodily sensation are also found. Patients complain of being vibrated, raped or forced to have sexual intercourse. Olfactory hallucinations often relating to poisonous gas are encountered. Visual hallucinations are rarer and, if present, should raise a suspicion of an underlying organic state. Patients are much less likely to have negative features than those who developed early onset schizophrenia and therefore have relatively good preservation of personality.

Management

The initial management of late-life psychosis involves evaluation and engagement. Patients are usually best assessed at home (rather than in a clinic) both because they are unlikely to comply with outpatient appointments and because their psychopathology may be strongly triggered by cues within their normal environment and less obvious when away from it. Health workers may initially find it difficult to gain access to the home of a patient with late-onset schizophrenia. Once initial access is gained, patients are often glad to gain a new audience for the expression of their delusional beliefs. Attempts at treatment should begin in the community wherever possible, with hospital admission reserved for patients with particularly severe or dangerous behavioural disturbance or poor self-care.

An attempt should be made to correct remediable physical or environmental contributory factors, particularly through alleviating sensory and/or social isolation. A flexible approach is required, and the patients' characteristic insistence on remaining isolated (as they have often been for much of their lives) must be respected. Patients' importuning requests for re-housing may be secondary to delusional beliefs and, if so, should be resisted. Although symptoms improve or even abate in a new home setting, this is usually a temporary respite. Old 'tormentors' re-emerge and new ones may be acquired. Anti-psychotic medication is a vital component of the total therapeutic package but is far from the whole answer. Improvisation, tenacity and ingenuity in engaging these patients and then retaining them in long-term follow-up are crucial to maintain both compliance and an optimal level of social functioning, and to reduce risk of symptomatic relapse.

Principles of drug treatment of psychotic illness (Box 25)

Dosages of neuroleptics are much lower than those used in younger patients with schizophrenia because older people with paraphrenia are often very sensitive to side effects. Each patient should ideally be prescribed only one anti-psychotic (except when switching from one to another). Anti-psychotics should be used to treat psychosis rather than as short-term sedation. If patients are very agitated or anxious, they can be given benzodiazepines in the short term while the anti-psychotics 'kick-in', which is less likely to cause long-term side effects. The lowest possible dose of anti-psychotics should be given and it should be prescribed preferably in a single dose, or at least in as few doses daily as possible given the properties of the drug. Compliance is a major problem in these patients, who usually live alone and do not have any insight into treatment necessity. Even when compliance is assured, many patients remain psychotic, although they may be less distressed by their symptoms and less disturbed in their behaviour. Community psychiatric nurses administering depot preparations may be more likely to ensure a favourable response but side effects are also likely to be greater.

> Box 25 General principles of prescribing anti-psychotics.
>
> - Prescribe one anti-psychotic at one time
> - Do not use for sedation
> - Use lowest possible dose
> - Use simplest possible regimen
> - Use caution with anticholinergic drugs

Anticholinergic drugs should not be given prophylactically. If patients develop extrapyramidal effects that require treatment with anticholinergic drugs, they should be withdrawn slowly once the patient has had 2 or 3 months free of side effects. They are drugs of misuse because they cause a 'buzz' and impair memory.

Considerations when using anti-psychotics in older people

The tolerability of all anti-psychotic drugs is affected by the higher rates of co-morbidity found in older people, the interaction with other drugs prescribed for other morbidities (see Chapter 3) and the increased susceptibility to side effects. As for antidepressants (see Chapter 2), the age-related changes in the renal, gastrointestinal and cardiac systems mean that most drugs are metabolized more slowly, and there is a greater fraction of active non-protein-bound drug available. Plasma concentrations vary hugely between older patients and this unpredictability is much more pronounced than in younger patients. In general, anti-psychotics need to be given at lower dosages. The general adage is 'start low and go slow'.

Conventional anti-psychotics

As conventional or typical anti-psychotics have been used since the 1950s, a considerable amount is known about their efficacy and their side effects. Conventional anti-psychotics are all antagonists of dopamine receptors. They are also cheap. In general, they have five main categories of side effects (*Box 26*). The side-effect profiles of typical anti-psychotics vary according to receptor occupancy of the different chemical structures and are set out in *Table 8*. The extrapyramidal side effects are mediated by D_2-receptor blockade in the nigrostriatal pathways, and one of the differences between the typical (conventional) anti-psychotics and the newer ones is their greater propensity to produce extrapyramidal side effects. Older people are much more sensitive to typical anti-psychotics and in particular are more likely to have early extrapyramidal side effects. The incidence of tardive dyskinesia is 5% year on year using the anti-psychotics listed in *Table 8*. The incidence is increased in older people, those with the emergence of early extrapyramidal symptoms and those with organic brain damage. Typical anti-psychotics should therefore be used with prudence in older people. They should generally be used only when there is a specific reason, e.g. the patient has responded in the past to a particular drug without side effects or is currently doing well on them. Another reason to use conventional anti-psychotics in older people is when depot medication is necessary because there are no depot atypical anti-psychotics at the time of writing. This situation is expected to change in the next few months.

Depot anti-psychotics

Depot anti-psychotics are long lasting. This means that adverse as well as therapeutic effects are likely to be long lasting. They are used when either the patient prefers them or, more commonly, when the mental health team believe that the patient is unlikely to comply with oral

---

Box 26 Categories of side effects of typical anti-psychotics.

- Extrapyramidal:
    immediate: acute dystonia
    short term: parkinsonism and akisthesia
    long term: tardive dyskinesia
- Hyperprolactinaemia:
    impotence
    amenorrhoea
    galactorrhoea
- Anti-adrenergic: postural hypotension
- Anticholinergic:
    dry mouth
    constipation
    urinary retention
    glaucoma
- Histaminic – sedation

Table 8 Typical anti-psychotic drugs: name, dose range, adverse effects, interactions.

Drug	Dose range (mg)	Adverse effects	Interactions	Special notes
Chlorpromazine	25–100	EPSEs, anticholinergic effects, sedation, hypotension, hypothermia, galactorrhoea, convulsions, idiosyncratic jaundice, blood dyscrasia, ECG changes	Sedatives, lithium, anticholinergics, anti-epileptics, sulphonylureas, cimetidine, dopamine agonists	High hypotensive effects
Promazine	200–400	As chlorpromazine	As chlorpromazine	Weak anti-psychotics
Thioridazine	25–400	As chlorpromazine, retinitis pigmentosa, ejaculatory dysfunction	As chlorpromazine	No longer to be prescribed
Fluphenazine	1–10	As chlorpromazine and depression	As chlorpromazine	High EPSEs
Perphenazine	6–12	As chlorpromazine	As chlorpromazine	High EPSEs
Trifluoperazine	5–25	As chlorpromazine	As chlorpromazine	High EPSEs
Flupenthixol	3–9	As chlorpromazine	As chlorpromazine	

Table 8 continued

Drug	Dose range (mg)	Adverse effects	Interactions	Special notes
Zuclopenthixol	10–75	As chlorpromazine	As chlorpromazine	
Haloperidol	0.5–20	As chlorpromazine	As chlorpromazine and fluoxetine	high EPSEs
Droperidol	10–40	As chlorpromazine and depression	As chlorpromazine	Used only for acute sedation
Benperidol	0.25–1.5	As chlorpromazine	As chlorpromazine	Used to decrease sex drive; not licensed as anti-psychotic
Pimozide	1–10	As chlorpromazine + serious cardiac arrhythmias (monitor potassium) and depression	As chlorpromazine and diuretics and cardioactive drugs, including tricyclic antidepressants and other anti-psychotics	ECG monitoring required

EPSEs, extrapyramidal side effects

Box 27 Principles of depot administration.

- Give a test dose
- Begin with the lowest possible dose
- Administer at the longest possible licensed interval
- Adjust dose only after adequate assessment

drugs. In the community, the patient must agree to have the drug. The principles of administration of depot anti-psychotics are shown in *Box 27*.

The first dose of depot anti-psychotic should be a test dose using the smallest possible dose to check that the patient can tolerate the drug. Once it has been started, the lowest possible therapeutic dose should be given. There is evidence that lower dosages are at least as effective as higher dosages, and patients should be on the minimum dose to control their symptoms. All depot anti-psychotics can safely be given at their longest licensed intervals and this is more pleasant for the patient because few people enjoy receiving an injection. As depot drugs may take time to reach steady-state and peak plasma levels, the dosage should be adjusted only some time after the patient has been started on the preparation.

Atypical anti-psychotics

Several definitions of what makes an anti-psychotic atypical have been proposed and some drugs can fall into the category of typical or atypical depending on the definition used. One definition is that atypical anti-psychotics are selective in dopamine blockade and another that they have greater potency for antagonizing serotonin $5HT_{2A}$-receptors than D_2-receptors. The former definition includes sulpiride and amisulpiride but the latter does not. All definitions include clozapine, risperidone, quetiapine and olanzapine.

Atypical anti-psychotics are recommended for people who cannot tolerate typical anti-psychotics. They are also recommended as first-line therapy for patients who are at high risk of extrapyramidal side effects and for those with first episode psychosis by NICE (National Institute of Clinical Excellence). This would clearly include many older people with late-onset schizophrenia and those with co-morbid Parkinson's disease or dementia (see Chapter 7). Some would argue that it would include all older people. The cost consideration is one that inhibits prescription of atypical anti-psychotics to everybody with a psychotic illness. Atypical anti-psychotics are also thought to be useful for the negative symptoms of schizophrenia. Sulpiride is currently the cheapest of the atypical anti-psychotics and, as a result of this, it should perhaps be the first-line therapy except in those people with parkinsonian symptoms. The drug that is theoretically least likely to cause extrapyramidal side effects is quetiapine, which is therefore the drug of choice for those with Parkinson's disease and a psychotic illness. The names, dosages, adverse effects and interactions of the atypical anti-psychotics are shown in *Table 9*. Their role in the treatment of psychosis in dementia is reviewed in Chapter 7.

Clozapine

Clozapine is the only drug that is recommended for refractory schizophrenia (defined as schizophrenia unresponsive to at least two adequate trials of antipsychotics, including an atypical). It is difficult to use because of its rare but potentially life-threatening side effect of agranulocytosis. Other side effects (hypersalivation, reduced seizure threshold, sedation) also limit its use. This means that the patient must be registered with the clozapine monitoring service and agree to regular venepuncture (weekly for the first 16 weeks) because the tablets will not be released unless the patient's white cell count is known to be satisfactory. The average dose used by all patients in the UK is 450 mg. It has many side effects and they tend to be worse in older people. Many of clozapine's adverse effects are dose dependent and are probably related to a rapid increase in dosage, especially at the beginning of therapy. It should be started at a dose of 12.5 mg daily and after the first dose blood pressure should be monitored hourly for the first 6 hours. Titration should be according to the response of the patient and the dose should be reduced if the patient becomes sedated or hypotensive and increased again more slowly.

Table 9 Names, dosages, side effects and interactions of the atypical drugs.

Drug	Dose range (mg)	Adverse effects	Interactions	Special notes
Sulpiride	200–1200	As chlorpromazine – EPSEs, anticholinergic effects, sedation, hypotension, hypothermia, galactorrhoea, convulsions, idiosyncratic jaundice, blood dyscrasia, ECG changes	Sedatives, lithium, anticholinergics, anti-epileptics, sulphonylureas, cimetidine, dopamine agonists	Jaundice, sedation, hypotension and EPSEs less common than chlorpromazine. Needs to be given twice daily
Risperidone	0.5–8	Agitation, hypotension, abdominal pain, fatigue, anxiety, nausea, rhinitis, weight gain, EPSEs	As sulpiride and quinidine	EPSEs uncommon at dosages < 2.0 mg
Olanzapine	5–20	Sedation, weight gain, hypotension, anticholinergic effects, hyperglycaemia, changes in LFTs, EPSEs	Theophylline, carbamazepine, digoxin and smoking reduce olanzapine levels	Blood glucose should be monitored before and after treatment started; EPSEs rare

Table 9 *continued.*

Drug	Dose range (mg)	Adverse effects	Interactions	Special notes
Quetiapine	100–500	Hypotension, sedation, dry mouth, constipation, weight gain, dizziness, LFT changes, TFT changes	Phenytoin. Caution with ketonacozole, nefazodone.	Needs to be given twice daily Theoretically no more EPSEs than placebo
Clozapine	25–900	As sulpiride + hypersalivation, delirium, incontinence, myocarditis, neutropenia, agranulocytis Reduced seizure threshold (as other anti-psychotics but particularly so)	As sulpiride and all drugs that suppress leukopoesis, e.g. cytotoxics and SSRIs (except citalopram), theophylline, digoxin, warfarin	Only drug recommended for resistant schizophrenia Monitoring required (see text). Blood glucose should also be monitored

EPSEs, extrapyramidal side effects; FTs, liver function tests; SSRIs, selective serotonin reuptake inhibitors; TFT, thyroid function test.

Dosage titration schedules that have been suggested for younger adults are likely to be too rapid for older adults who will also probably respond to lower dosages. As with the other anti-psychotics, there are no placebo-controlled trials in older people with schizophrenia. There is, however, a report of clozapine in 329 older patients with refractory psychosis (aged > 55 years) which found a good response, particularly for positive symptoms. The results of a trial comparing clozapine with placebo in the treatment of psychosis in Parkinson's disease also finds that it significantly improves the symptoms without worsening the psychosis, and again it may be a useful drug for those patients refractory to or intolerant of treatment with the other atypical anti-psychotics.

Overall clozapine is efficacious but poorly tolerated in older people. The major side effect of agranulocytosis increases with age. It should be used only in those patients in whom other treatments have proved ineffective or intolerable, and who remain significantly distressed or a risk to themselves or others.

chapter 7

Anti-dementia drugs

The dementia syndrome (progressive global cognitive impairment) can be seen as a final common symptom pathway for several distinct disease entities, of which the most common are Alzheimer's disease (AD), vascular dementia (VaD) and dementia with Lewy bodies (DLB). Early studies of drug treatments for the cognitive symptoms of the dementias examined their efficacy in mixed cohorts. More recently, specific treatments have been and are being evaluated for each of these common dementias, with particular emphasis being placed on possible treatments for AD. Although the early emphasis was on treatments that affected cognition, later trials have considered both cognition and other domains such as activity of daily living skills. Both for the dementias as a whole and for AD in particular, treatment approaches can be classified as preventive, disease modifying and symptomatic.

Disease prevention

Preventive approaches in Alzheimer's disease
As the pathological changes in AD start years and possibly decades before symptoms are obvious, the rational approach to the disease is to start to use preventive approaches for those at high risk before development of symptoms.

The prevention of AD can be attempted in several ways. The most direct approach is genetic. Further preventive strategies in AD involve the use of antioxidants, anti-inflammatory drugs and hormones.

Genetic approaches

As our understanding of the genetic basis of the disease increases, the prospects for specific gene therapies improve. Several specific genetic markers for AD have now been identified. They usually act at some stage of the amyloid cascade system. The increase in amyloid is related to tau phosphorylation but it is not clear if it induces it. Some are rare but occur in affected members of families with high rates of early onset AD, and may directly cause the increase in amyloid deposition in the brain by preventing the breakdown of amyloid precursor protein (APP). Others (most notably the E4 variant of the apolipoprotein E gene on chromosome 19) are commonly found in people with late-onset AD. As yet no specific gene-modifying treatments have been fully evaluated.

The AD vaccine has come from immunizing transgenic animals. These animals have been bred with the mutation that causes increased APP to be synthesized. When amyloid was injected into these animals, they developed an immune response and the number of plaques decreased. Trials are at present taking place in humans, although recently there have been reports that some people have not tolerated the experimental treatment. Nevertheless, this treatment still offers hope for the future and is the only treatment that has been observed to decrease the neuropathology.

Antioxidants

There is increasing evidence that AD is associated with reduced activity, within the brain, of naturally occurring antioxidants (such as superoxide dismutase), resulting in the generation of free radicals and increased vulnerability to oxidative damage to neurons. Amyloid itself may generate free radicals. Several antioxidant chemicals have been suggested as potentially useful in protecting against or modifying AD pathology, including vitamin C, vitamin E and the traditional Chinese remedy *Gingko biloba*. There is some evidence that vitamin E postpones deterioration in established AD with increasing time, until the patient has to be admitted to a nursing home. The doses were, however, huge and very much more than in dietary supplements, which are unlikely to have any antioxidant effects. Trials of *Gingko biloba* show that it may cause limited cognitive improvement. None of these substances is as yet licensed for the treatment or prevention of AD.

Anti-inflammatories

The inflammatory process (both in the brain and peripherally) can induce the formation of amyloid peptides. Inflammation may thus be linked to the deposition of amyloid plaques, one of the characteristic pathological findings in the AD brain. Most naturalistic case–control studies suggest that elderly people who regularly take high doses of non-steroidal anti-inflammatory drugs (NSAIDs) have a reduced risk of developing AD. There are no randomized double-masked trials of NSAIDs and none is as yet licensed for the treatment or prevention of AD.

Hormones

Oestrogens have several actions that may be preventive or disease modifying in AD, including promotion of the breakdown of amyloid precursor protein, antioxidant effects and the facilitation of cholinergic neurotransmission. Several epidemiological studies suggest that women on hormone replacement therapy are at substantially (35–50%) reduced risk of developing AD. There are 10 randomized trials of hormone treatment, of which three found significant improvements in memory and two in attention. Higher doses (≥ 1.25 mg) may confer greater protection than lower (≤ 0.625 mg) doses. Co-administered progestins may reduce the protective effect. There are no comparative data on different oestrogen preparations and none suggesting therapeutic benefits for oestrogens in men. Oestrogens are not as yet licensed for the treatment or prevention of AD.

Lithium

Phosphorylated tau (τ) binds to itself, making the neurofibrillary tangles of AD (and some other dementias). Tau is phosphorylated by an enzyme called GSK-3 (glycogen synthase kinase 3β), which is inhibited by lithium in vivo and in rats. This reduces tau phosphorylation and restores tau's normal function in the neuron.

Preventing VaD

Preventive strategies for VaD involve identifying those at high risk and attempting to modify specific risk factors. The risk factors for VaD are essentially the same as risk factors for stroke and include hypertension, hyperlipidaemia, diabetes, smoking and obesity. Probably the best markers of high risk of VaD are a history of stroke or transient ischaemic attacks (TIAs). Smoking cessation and optimal control of specific risk factors such as hypertension, particularly high systolic blood pressure, may be effective in both preventing the establishment of VaD and slowing its progression. Exercise has been shown to decrease progression of cognitive impairment, although this may not be specific for VaD. Statins may be useful in reducing risk of stroke (and by extension VaD) even in the absence of clear-cut hyperlipidaemia. Detailed information on their use is beyond the scope of this chapter and the reader is advised to consult the *British National Formulary*.

The most widely used drug treatments for those at high risk of or with established VaD are aspirin and dipyridamole, which exert an anti-thrombolytic effect by modifying platelet aggregation, adhesion and survival. The use of these anti-platelet agents is contraindicated in haemorrhagic stroke. The Cochrane review of the use of aspirin in dementia commented that aspirin was a rational study because it inhibits platelet aggregation and 80% of patients with VaD in UK are prescribed aspirin. Long-term aspirin to those with a history of TIAs or ischaemic stroke decrease fatal cerebrovascular accidents by 20% and decrease non-fatal ones by one-third; there is no evidence at all of its efficacy or otherwise in VaD.

Aspirin 75–150 mg/day is probably as effective as higher doses and carries less risk of inducing gastrointestinal bleeding. Dipyridamole may be used alone in patients in whom aspirin is contraindicated, or together with aspirin. It is thought that the effects of aspirin and dipyridamole on platelet activity are additive. The dose range for dipyridamole is between 300 and 600 mg/day, in divided doses. A sustained release formulation (200 mg twice daily) is now also available. Dipyridamole may increase the hypotensive effect of blood pressure-lowering drugs and may reduce the activity of cholinesterase inhibitors.

Disease-modifying treatments

Box 28 shows the effects that a disease-modifying drug might have. Future developments for modifying the progression of AD are likely to include modulators of protein processing – in particular preventing or removing deposits of amyloid and/or tau proteins (the main constituents of senile plaques and neurofibrillary tangles, respectively). Oestrogens and cholinesterase inhibitors may have limited activity in this area and more specific modulators are currently being developed.

Meanwhile several drugs have been shown to have activity in protecting neurons against damage and/or to stimulate neuronal growth. These may be beneficial in both AD and VaD.

So-called 'nootropic' drugs have been advocated for the treatment of AD and other dementias such as VaD. They were originally thought to exert their therapeutic action by inducing cerebral vasodilatation. In this

Box 28 Possible effects of disease modification in dementia.

- Cognition improves
- Cognition stable
- Cognition deteriorates more slowly
- Independence preserved
- Reversal of disease process
- Slowing of disease process
- Reduction of costs of caring in the short term
- Reduction of carer burden in the short term
- Reduction of excess mortality
- Increased survival time with disease at any stage

model, dementia is seen as resulting from 'cerebrovascular insufficiency' and thereby potentially treatable by inducing such cerebral vasodilatation. Unfortunately, even in VaD, vasodilatation does not cause a beneficial redistribution of blood supply to ischaemic brain tissue. The longest established of this group of drugs are the ergot derivatives, of which the most widely used is Hydergine (co-dergocrine maleate). Hydergine is currently classified as a 'metabolic enhancer' and there is little specific evidence for its efficacy; it may exert some neuroprotective effect in both AD and VaD. Some trials, however, suggest that it may be harmful. The usual daily dose is 4.5 mg, in single or divided doses. Piracetam 800–100 mg daily is another 'nootropic', although dementia is not as yet an indication for its use.

The monoamine oxidase (MAO) B inhibitor selegiline has been shown to postpone deterioration significantly in established AD. Selegiline at the usual dose of 10 mg/day is sufficiently MAO-B selective not to require a low tyramine diet. It is rapidly absorbed after oral administration and has several active metabolites, including metamphetamine. Adverse interactions may occur with pethidine and with SSRI (selective serotonin reuptake inhibitor) antidepressants. AD and VaD are not as yet recognized indications for the use of selegiline.

The xanthine derivative propentofylline is likely to be licensed soon for the treatment of VaD and AD. Propentofylline exerts a neuroprotective effect through inhibition of adenosine reuptake and phosphodiesterase activity (thus reducing cyclic AMP degradation). In addition it reduces microglial activation and resultant neuronal damage. Propentofylline has been shown to improve cerebral glucose metabolism in patients with AD and in those with acute stroke. Most clinical studies have been in mixed AD and VaD samples. Benefits are seen in cognitive and global measures, with most studies suggesting more impressive benefits in VaD. The dose of propentofylline in most studies is 300 mg three times a day. The drug is generally well tolerated although gastrointestinal disturbances, dizziness and headache are sometimes experienced.

Nicotine

Acetylcholine stimulates muscarinic and nicotinic receptors. There is a profound loss of nicotinic receptors, although muscarinic ones remain virtually unchanged in AD. There is controversial evidence that smoking may be protective in AD with contradictory studies. The Cochrane review of the subject found only one study of nicotine for AD with eight people in it and concluded that there was no evidence of efficacy.

Symptomatic treatments

More recently, interest has focused on AD as a distinct disease entity, and within AD research on drugs with specific activity on the cholinergic neurotransmitter system. These treatments have their basis in the observation that at the neurotransmitter level the most pervasive deficit in AD is a reduction in levels of acetylcholine resulting from loss of cholinergic neurons (the cell bodies of which are in the nucleus basalis of Meynert). Postsynaptic cholinergic receptors are relatively well preserved. It is important to remember, however, that many other neurotransmitter deficits (as well as gross neuronal loss and reduction in dendritic branching) are also found in AD, and that one would therefore not expect cholinergic 'boosting' to reverse all the cognitive and behavioural deficits.

Initial trials of acetylcholine precursors (choline and lecithin) were disappointing. In contrast, cholinesterase inhibitors showed greater early promise, which has been confirmed in several large clinical trials. As a result, four cholinesterase inhibitors (tacrine, donepezil, galantamine and rivastigmine) are currently licensed for the symptomatic treatment of mild-to-moderate AD and several more such drugs have received extensive clinical trial evaluation. These include metrifonate (an organophosphate long used for the treatment of schistosomiasis), velnacrine, slow-release physostigmine and eptastigmine (a pro-drug of physostigmine). In general, cholinesterase inhibitors produce modest but statistically significant improvements or prevent deterioration in cognitive function, with some studies of some drugs also suggesting benefits in global functioning, daily living skills and carer burden. Degree of change varies greatly between individuals. In the light of this and of the nature of AD as a chronically progressive condition, mean change scores in randomized controlled trials provide less clinically useful information than is usually the case. Analyses of number needed to treat (NNT) (see Chapter 2), however, reveal NNTs between 4 and 7 for several clinically meaningful indices of individual response, and suggest that these drugs may be clinically useful and even cost-effective. Long-term data are still lacking, but available evidence suggests that typical responses are of the order of a 6- to 12-month reversal or postponement of deterioration, with a minority of patients maintaining a more sustained improvement. There is also some suggestion that long-term use of cholinesterase inhibitors may delay disease progression in AD.

There has, to date, been little formal study of symptomatic treatments in DLB. Cholinesterase inhibitors are probably effective, particularly in alleviating psychotic symptoms. Dopaminergic treatments have proved disappointing.

Particularly during the first few years of clinical experience with these drugs, they should be prescribed within a locally agreed protocol. The main features of such a protocol are outlined below. Cholinesterase inhibitors should be used only in patients in whom there is a clear diagnosis of AD, with documentation that patients meet standard criteria such as those of ICD-10 (*International Classification of Diseases*, 5th edn) or DSM-IV (*Diagnostic and Statistical Manual of Mental Disorders*, 4th edn). The efficacy of this group of drugs has only been shown for the sub-group of AD patients with mild to moderately severe AD (Mini Mental State scores of 10–26 or, in the case of rivastigmine, which has been tested in a wider range of patients, 6–26). Patients and their carers should have the side effects and possible benefits of the drugs explained to them and issues of consent and compliance (which may require carer support) considered. Titration to optimal dose will require close initial monitoring. Clinician and carer (and where possible patients themselves) should monitor progress closely, with a decision taken after 3–6 months of treatment about whether continuation of the drug is justified. Such justification will usually involve improvement (or at least lack of deterioration) in at least two areas of functioning. Areas to be considered can include cognition, global functioning, mood, daily living skills, behaviour and carer burden. The initial prescription should be following specialist referral and assessment, and specialist involvement in the decision to continue is also helpful. Rapid deterioration may occur after drug discontinuation (even where there has been little or no apparent benefit during treatment); this may be reversed following re-establishment of treatment.

Choice of drug

The choice of drug is governed by efficacy, ease of administration, tolerability and cost (see Chapter 2). Patients with AD are often frail and, by the nature of the disease, find it difficult to remember to take drugs. They often need to be reminded by the carer, who may be family or statutory services. The burden of care on the carer or the cost of the statutory services, as well as of the drug itself, therefore governs the choice. A final consideration is the ease of reaching the correct dosage. The drugs that require more titration may be a much greater burden to the patient, the carer and the doctor. *Tables 10–13* compare the efficacy and tolerability of donepezil, rivastigmine, tacrine and galantamine, for different endpoints in terms of NNTs and numbers needed to harm (NNHs) (see Chapter 2 for more details of NNTs).

Tacrine was the first cholinesterase inhibitor to complete the clinical trial process and be licensed. It produces similar cognitive changes to those found with other cholinesterase inhibitors, but its clinical utility is severely limited by the high risk it carries of severe and sometimes irreversible hepatotoxicity. Tacrine is currently in use in the USA and some other countries. Although it has been licensed in the UK, it is not actively marketed and is unlikely to be widely used. Tacrine is 55% protein bound and extensively metabolized in the liver via the cytochrome P450 1A2 enzyme system. Tacrine may increase blood theophylline levels and its own plasma levels may be elevated by concomitant cimetidine. The initial recommended dose of tacrine is 10 mg four times daily, increasing by 40 mg/day (in four divided doses) every

Table 10 NNT for rivastigmine compared with placebo in AD.

Measure	Dose (mg)	No. of weeks	No. on placebo	No. on active	Percentage poor outcome (placebo)	Percentage poor outcome (active)	NNT (95% CI)
ADAS-COG: improvement ⩾ 4	1–4	26	239	242	84	85	−10 (−13–19)
CIBIC-Plus improvement	1–4	26	239	242	80	70	10.0 (6–44)
PDS (ADL): improvement > 10%	1–4	26	239	242	81	81	∞ (−14–15)
ADAS-COG: improvement ⩾ 4	6–12	26	239	243	84	76	13 (7–111)
CIBIC-Plus improvement	6–12	26	239	243	80	63	6 (4–11)
PDS (ADL): improvement > 10%	6–12	26	239	243	81	71	10 (6–42)
ADAS-COG: no deterioration	6–12	26	197	149	73	44	4 (3–6)
ADAS-COG: decline ⩾ 4	6–12	26	197	149	44	21	5 (3–8)

Table 10 *continued*.

Measure	Dose (mg)	No. of weeks	No. on placebo	No. on active	Percentage poor outcome (placebo)	Percentage poor outcome (active)	NNT (95% CI)
ADAS-COG: decline ⩾ 7	6–12	26	197	149	30	7	5 (4–7)
CIBIC-Plus improvement	6–12	26	197	149	84	76	12.5 (−179–6)
CIBIC-Plus improvement	1–4	26	197	149	84	75	12 (6–273)
PDS (ADL): improvement > 10%	6–12	26	197	149	85	75	10 (6–70)

CI, confidence interval; ADAS-Cog, Alzheimer's Disease Assessment Scale (Cognitive subscale); CIBIC-Plus, Clinician's Interview Based Impression of Change Plus; MMSE, Mini Mental State Examination; PDS, Progressive Deterioration Scale; ADL, activities of daily living; NA, not applicable as patients not improved on this outcome measure by the drug.

Table 11 NNT for donepezil compared with placebo in AD.

Measure	Dose (mg)	No. of weeks	No. on placebo	No. on active	Percentage poor outcome (placebo)	Percentage poor outcome (active)	NNT (95% CI)
ADAS-COG: no deterioration	5	24	153	152	42	20	5 (4–9)
ADAS-COG: improvement ⩾ 4	5	24	153	152	73	62	10 (5–180)
ADAS-COG: improvement ⩾ 7	5	24	153	152	92	85	15 (−828–8)
ADAS-COG: no deterioration	10	24	153	150	42	19	5 (3–8)
ADAS-COG: improvement ⩾ 4	10	24	153	150	73	47	4 (3–7)
ADAS-COG: improvement ⩾ 7	10	24	153	150	92	75	6 (4–12)
CIBIC-Plus improvement ⩾ 3	5	24	152	149	89	74	7 (5–16)

Table 11 *continued.*

Measure	Dose (mg)	No. of weeks	No. on placebo	No. on active	Percentage poor outcome (placebo)	Percentage poor outcome (active)	NNT (95% CI)
CIBIC-Plus deterioration ⩾ 5	5	24	152	149	45	33	9 (5–94)
CIBIC-Plus improvement ⩾ 3	10	24	152	149	89	75	8 (5–19)
CIBIC-Plus deterioration ⩾ 5	10	24	152	149	45	25	5 (4–11)

CI, confidence interval; ADAS-Cog, Alzheimer's Disease Assessment Scale (Cognitive subscale); CIBIC-Plus, Clinician's Interview Based Impression of Change Plus.

Table 12 NNT for tacrine compared with placebo in AD.

Measure	Dose (mg)	No. of weeks	No. on placebo	No. on active	Percentage poor outcome (placebo)	Percentage poor outcome (active)	NNT (95% CI)
CIBI improvt	160	30	116	64	82	58	5 (4–11)
ADAS-Cog improvt ≥ 4	160	30	116	64	75	60	7 (3–10)
MMSE improvt ≥ 3	160	30	116	64	80	58	5 (4–156)

CI, confidence interval; ADAS-Cog, Alzheimer's Disease Assessment Scale (Cognitive subscale); CIBIC-Plus, Clinician's Interview Based Impression of Change Plus; MMSE, Mini Mental State Examination, improvt, improvement.

Table 13 NNT for galantamine compared with placebo in AD.

Measure	Dose (mg)	No. of weeks	No. on placebo	No. on active	Percentage poor outcome (placebo)	Percentage poor outcome (active)	NNT (95% CI)
CIBI no change or improvt	24	30	213	212	44.7	29.6	8 (4–56)
ADAS-Cog improvt ⩾ 4	24	30	213	212	83.4	67.7	6 (4–14)
Discontinuation	24	30	213	212	8	23	7 (5–12)
CIBI no change or improvt	32	30	213	211	44.7	32.1	8 (4–71)
ADAS-Cog improvt ⩾ 4	32	30	213	211	83.4	67.4	6 (4–14)
Discontinuation	32	30	213	211	8	32	4 (3–6)

CI, confidence interval; ADAS-Cog, Alzheimer's Disease Assessment Scale (Cognitive subscale); CIBIC-Plus, Clinician's Interview Based Impression of Change Plus; MMSE, Mini Mental State Examination. improvt, improvement.

6 weeks to a maximum of 40 mg four times daily. Liver function needs to be monitored carefully in patients taking tacrine and becomes abnormal in about 50% of patients on the drug. Weekly blood testing is necessary for the first 18 weeks, with further testing every 3 months if liver function remains normal. The drug should be discontinued if transaminase levels increase by more than three- to five-fold. The development of jaundice mandates immediate withdrawal of tacrine. Other tacrine side effects are similar to those described for donepezil below (but are more frequently observed). These side effects reflect enhanced cholinergic function.

Donepezil is a specific and reversible inhibitor of acetylcholinesterase. It is well absorbed by mouth, with peak plasma concentrations after 3–4 hours. Donepezil has a half-life of about 3 days. Steady-state plasma concentrations are reached after 2–3 weeks. Donepezil is highly (95%) protein bound, and is partly excreted intact in the urine and partly metabolized in the liver through the cytochrome P450 system. Donepezil is given in a single daily dose, preferably in the evening. It is the only licensed cholinesterase inhibitor that can be given in a single dose. The starting dose is 5 mg. Side effects permitting, the dose can be increased after 4 weeks to 10 mg with the possibility of increased efficacy but a greater risk of side effects. The most frequent side effects are gastrointestinal (diarrhoea and muscle cramps). Other side effects include fatigue, nausea, vomiting, insomnia and dizziness. No important drug interactions have been demonstrated, although there is potential for interference with anticholinergic medications (which should in any case be avoided in patients with AD) and potentiation of depolarizing neuromuscular blockers (such as suxamethonium) or cholinergic agonists. Overdosage may result in a 'cholinergic crisis' characterized by nausea, vomiting, salivation, sweating, bradycardia, hypotension and respiratory collapse. Treatment is with atropine and supportive measures.

Rivastigmine is a carbamate derivative which binds to and temporarily inactivates acetylcholinesterase. Peak plasma concentrations occur one hour after oral ingestion. Rivastigmine is weakly (40%) protein bound and is rapidly and extensively metabolized primarily via extrahepatic cholinesterase-mediated hydrolysis. Enzyme activity normalizes about 9 hours after a single dose. Rivastigmine should be given twice daily. The initial recommended dose is 1.5 mg twice daily. If tolerated, this can be increased after 2 weeks to 3 mg twice daily and (after further 2-week periods) to 4.5 mg twice daily, and thence to the maximum recommended dose of 6 mg twice daily. The main side effects described are nausea, vomiting, abdominal pain, loss of appetite, asthenia and somnolence. Other side effects (which are closely related to speed of dose titration) include sweating, malaise, weight loss and tremor. Unlike donepezil, rivastigmine clearance is not affected by impaired renal or hepatic function. Rivastigmine has a low propensity for adverse drug interactions. The management of rivastigmine overdosage is similar to that described for donepezil above.

Galantamine is a competitive inhibitor of acetylcholinesterase and a nicotinic receptor agonist. Its modulatory effect on nicotinic receptors potentiates the response of these receptors to acetyl cholinesterase. It was originally produced from the snowdrop family of flowers, but is now produced synthetically. It has a relatively short half-life of 5.5 hours and so needs to be given twice daily.

Cholinesterase inhibitors and drug interactions

There is, as yet, relatively little research evidence concerning interactions between the cholinesterase inhibitors and other drugs. The most important effects noted to date are increased cholinergic side effects where these drugs are given in combination with the SSRI fluvoxamine or the antifungal ketoconazole. In both cases this probably reflects drug-induced cytochrome P450 3A3/4 inhibition. Rivastigmine has been found to be relatively free of adverse interactions when given in combination with a wide range of therapeutic classes of drugs, including antacids, benzodiazepines, NSAIDs and antihypertensives. This suggests that (as might be expected in terms of its minimal metabolism by cytochrome P450 enzymes) rivastigmine is the safest of the currently available cholinesterase inhibitors in terms of potential for adverse interactions.

chapter 8

Behavioural and psychiatric symptoms of dementia

What are the behavioural and psychiatric symptoms of dementia?

Although the cognitive impairments in dementia are the defining and perhaps most easily measurable aspects of the disease, there are many other symptoms and signs that collectively are known as behavioural and psychiatric symptoms of dementia (BPSD). Changes in the ability to function and in cognition cluster together and therefore seem to be symptoms of the same underlying pathology. These are not mirrored by changes in BPSD, which is now seen as a distinct syndrome that should be considered independently of the cognitive and functional domains of the dementing process. There are many symptoms in this cluster. A list of some of the common individual symptoms of BPSD is given in *Box 29*.

How common are BPSDs?

The only epidemiological study of BPSD in people with dementia in the community showed that 60% of individuals with AD reported at least one symptom, a third of those with BPSD had multiple symptoms.

In clinical practice, BPSD affects about 80% of those referred to psychiatric services. *Table 14* shows the prevalence in two clinical populations,

Box 29 BPSD of dementia.

Psychiatric symptoms	Behavioural symptoms
Delusions	Aggression
Hallucinations	Wandering
Anxiety	Inappropriate motor activity
Apathy	Sleep disturbance
Phobias	Disinhibition
Misrecognition	Hyperorality or loss of appetite
Anger	

the first of whom all had AD and the second all types of dementia. It is notable, but unsurprising, that people with dementia who have been referred to a psychiatrist have much higher rates of BPSDs. The most common symptoms were angry outbursts, paranoid symptoms, and dietary and sleeping changes.

Dementia with Lewy bodies (DLB) is a form of dementia in which visual hallucinations early in the illness are particularly common. As they are one of the symptoms listed in the consensus diagnostic criteria, two out of three of which must be present to make the diagnosis, many if not most patients with this disorder have hallucinations at some point in the illness. People with DLB are also likely to suffer from sensitivity to conventional neuroleptics and this means that there are particular problems in treating this group of patients (see below).

The importance of BPSD

As well as the distress that can be caused to the patient by BPSD, these symptoms can also impact greatly on the mental health of the carer. Caring for people with such difficulties is one of the main factors that has been associated with carer psychiatric morbidity. Thus, successful management of behavioural difficulties in a community setting may improve carer well-being. In addition, carer distress and depression are

Table 14 The range and frequency of BPSDs in referred patients with dementia.

	Behaviour frequency	
	Swearer et al (1988) No. (%)	Burns et al (1990) No. (%)
Angry outbursts	64 (51)	
Paranoia	40 (32)	
Paranoid delusions		10 (5.6)
Paranoid ideation		36 (20.2)
Dietary change	57 (46)	
Hyperorality		17 (9.8)
Binge eating		11 (6.3)
Sleep disturbance		55 (45)
Violent behaviour	27 (21)	35 (19.7)
Bizarre behaviour	26 (21)	
Hallucinations	28 (22)[a]	30 (16.9)
Delusions	28 (22)[a]	28 (16)
Misidentification		54 (30)
Phobia		31 (25)
Withdrawal/Apathy		71 (40.8)

[a] Swearer et al. included delusions and hallucinations in a single category, so the same figure of 22% refers to both together.

associated with the breakdown of care at home for people with dementia, and the requirement of 24-hour care within an institution.

Management of BPSD

Underlying additional pathology may be the cause of new symptoms in patients with dementia; they are vulnerable to deterioration in the form of BPSD when there is a new physical illness. This should be considered, as well as the possibility that these symptoms are an intrinsic feature of the dementia. All patients presenting with these symptoms for the first time therefore require an assessment of the cause. This should comprise: assessment of the possibility of iatrogenic causes, usually the prescription of new drugs; a physical examination, looking for signs and symptoms of infections and localizing neurological symptoms; and haematological investigations, including a screen for infection. Cerebral events and infection may present as BPSD, e.g. visual hallucinations, agitation or sleep disturbance. Pain and constipation may also lead to, for example, agitation or aggression and should be considered and looked for. Many BPSDs are treated with non-drug management, including environmental manipulation, increased activities and behavioural therapies.

Pharmacological treatment of BPSD

Drug treatment is also commonly employed for the BPSD but should be used sparingly, in low dosages and in conjunction with appropriate non-pharmacological treatment.

Drugs that increase serotonin for BPSD

Based on the theory that aggressive behaviour is mediated by the serotoninergic (5HT) system, drugs that act on this system have been tried for aggression in dementia. Trazodone, which has a 5HT reuptake blocking action, and buspirone, a 5HT agonist, have both been reported to be effective in controlling aggressive behaviour in patients with dementia. Citalopram and fluoxetine, selective 5HT-reuptake inhibitors (see Chapter 3) have been used successfully in the treatment of people with dementia who become agitated. Citalopram has also been effective in people who have disinhibition in the form of aggression or pathological tearfulness when the frontal lobe is involved. Carbamazepine has been found to be effective in treating aggression in dementia and this may be caused by its 5HT-enhancing activity or other activity (see below).

Anticonvulsants

Anticonvulsants have been used to treat BPSD as well as in mania (see details of the individual drugs in Chapter 5). One randomized controlled trial (RCT), which compared carbamazepine with placebo in 51 nursing home residents over a period of 6 weeks for BPSDs at a dose of 300 mg/day, found that it was significantly better than placebo. The changes were the result of decreased agitation and aggression rather than improvement in other symptoms. Withdrawal from the treatment for 3 weeks led to patients reverting to their baseline state. There was a variety of non-serious adverse effects, but no serious toxicity or death. Cognition remained steady, as did function.

Sodium valproate has been found to reduce BPSD in several studies. One report in patients with personality disorders found it effective in an open label study of non-responders to selective serotonin reuptake inhibitors (SSRIs) used for treating aggression.

A case report about use of gabapentin 300 mg three times daily in a patient whose BPSD had failed to respond to, or who had been unable to tolerate, antidepressants, neuroleptics or benzodiazepines found that it reduced agitation, sexual inappropriateness and lability.

Benzodiazepines

Benzodiazepines have also been found to be superior to placebo when used in the management of agitation and/or aggression in dementia. Oxazepam has also been found to be similar to haloperidol in one study for agitation and psychosis in dementia. However, they can have a paradoxical effect, such that they may worsen the agitation and/or aggression. They may also worsen cognitive impairment. Although they may be effective in the short term, tolerance to the sedative effects will occur but not to the amnesic effects. They should therefore always be used for a maximum period of 6 weeks and withdrawn slowly. They have also been used for sleep disturbance in dementia. Controlled trials of nitrazepam in patients with dementia show hangover effects, worsening of cognitive impairment and high rates of discontinuation. Relatively short-acting benzodiazepines are less likely to cause these problems.

Anti-psychotic treatment

Principles of use of anti-psychotics in BPSDs

Chapter 7 discusses in detail the anti-psychotics available and their effects in older people. People with dementia are particularly vulnerable to the side effects of anti-psychotic medication. They are more likely to suffer extrapyramidal side effects than those who are cognitively unimpaired. This population is at particular risk of developing tardive dyskinesia, although such movements can occur in those with dementia who have never received neuroleptics. The onset of dyskinesia may be more rapid than tardive dyskinesia.

As people with dementia tend to be in the very old age group, they usually have multiple pathology and drug interactions are therefore more frequently relevant (see Chapter 10). The co-morbidity means that, for example, cardiac side effects such as lengthening of the Q–T interval and postural hypotension are more probable. Sensitivity to anti-psychotic medication accompanied by cognitive decline has been documented in dementia in general. A 1997 study, involving a 2-year follow-up of 71 patients with dementia, found that the 16 who were taking typical anti-psychotic medications experienced twice the cognitive decline of those who were not taking them, as measured by the Mini Mental State Examination. This finding was independent of the behavioural problems for which the neuroleptics had been prescribed. The anti-psychotics used were all non-selective, the study was naturalistic and therefore it is unclear whether the control group was comparable, so no diagnosis of dementia subtype was made.

Neuroleptic sensitivity is a particular problem in DLB. This sensitivity takes the form of a much higher likelihood of extrapyramidal symptoms, a worsening of cognition, physical deterioration, immobility and increased death rate. This is particularly common with typical anti-psychotics, although it can also occur with the atypical ones. As quetiapine may not produce extrapyramidal effects, it is the rational first choice in this condition, although there are no published RCTs.

Haloperidol

The Cochrane review of haloperidol for BPSD of dementia found that agitated patients given haloperidol showed no improvement, in comparison to controls. They found some evidence that haloperidol helps to control aggression. Individual analysis of reports indicated that higher-dose haloperidol (> 2 mg/day) may have been more effective than lower-dose haloperidol (< 2 mg/day) in controlling aggression, but not of other manifestations of agitation, among patients with mild-to-moderate dementia. Drop-out rates were higher for haloperidol compared with placebo-treated patients, suggesting that side effects led to discontinuation of treatment in some patients.

One study compared haloperidol to oxazepam and diphenhydramine for agitation and psychosis and showed little difference in efficacy.

Higher-dose haloperidol, or prolonged haloperidol (> 2 mg for 12 weeks compared with 3–6 weeks), was associated with increased side effects, largely related to parkinsonian symptoms of rigidity and bradykinesia.

Thioridazine

The Cochrane review of thioridazine for BPSD of dementia concluded that, if thioridazine were not currently in widespread clinical use, there would be inadequate evidence to support its introduction. The only positive effect of thioridazine when compared with placebo was the reduction of anxiety. When compared with placebo, other neuroleptics and other sedatives, it had equal or higher rates of adverse effects. There is no evidence to support the use of thioridazine in dementia, and its use may expose patients to excess side effects. The Committee on Safety of Medicines has withdrawn thioridazine from use in the UK.

Depot anti-psychotics

There are case reports, but no trials, of very-low-dose depot anti-psychotic drugs being used to help with compliance in forgetful patients. This may have the advantage of ensuring more stable blood levels.

Comparison of anti-psychotic drugs

A naturalistic follow-up study of patients who had been prescribed haloperidol (289), olanzapine (209) and risperidone (500) for BPSDs in hospital found that, using the Brief Psychogeriatric Dependency Rating Scale, olanzapine was significantly superior to both risperidone and haloperidol in reducing aggression and delusions/hallucinations. In addition, olanzapine was significantly superior to risperidone in reducing noisiness and manipulative behaviour, which suggests olanzapine as the drug of choice in hospitalized patients with BPSD.

NNT analysis of RCTs for BPSD

Anti-psychotic efficacy in placebo-controlled trials

Table 15 shows the number needed to treat (NNT) and confidence intervals (CIs) for placebo-controlled studies of anti-psychotics in dementia. Olanzapine, risperidone 1–2 mg, haloperidol 0.25–4 mg and haloperidol 2–4 mg all had low NNTs with 95%CI values that did not include infinity. The trial of risperidone with a wider range of dosages (0.25–4 mg) was not significantly efficacious. In the trial of olanzapine, the dose was randomly allocated to 5 mg, 10 mg or 15 mg. The 5-mg dose of olanzapine was more efficacious than the 10-mg dose. The 15-mg dose had an even higher NNT and was not significantly more efficacious than placebo. Trifluoperazine and loxapine did not show evidence of efficacy.

Anti-psychotic efficacy in head-to-head anti-psychotic trials

There is no significant differences between any drugs used for BPSDs in head-to-head trials.

Adverse effects in placebo-controlled trials

Table 16 shows the number needed to harm (NNH) for placebo-controlled trials of anti-psychotics. Trifluoperazine 8 mg was the most likely to cause extrapyramidal side effects (EPSEs: NNH = 2, 95%CI = 1–9). Haloperidol 0.25–4 mg and 2–10 mg and risperidone 1–2 mg also had low and significant NNHs for EPSEs. None of the trials of olanzapine reported EPSEs. All doses of olanzapine caused somnolence, but the NNH fell as the dose increased. Risperidone 1–2 mg and 0.25–4 mg also caused somnolence. Non-specified adverse events were

Table 15 Numbers needed to treat for different antipsychotics for BPSD when compared with placebo.

Drugs (dosage)	Number of patients (drug 1, placebo)	Measure BPSD	Drug 1 (%)	Drug 2 (%)	NNT (95%CI)
Risperidone (0.25–4 mg)	115, 114	Behave -AD improvement by 30%	54	47	14 (5–∞)
Haloperidol (0.25–4 mg)	115, 114	Behave -AD improvement by 30%	63	47	6 (3–30)
Risperidone (1–2 mg)	313, 163	Behave -AD improvement by 30%	48	33	7 (4–17)
Olanzapine (5 mg)	56, 47	Neuropsychiatric Index	65.5	35.6	3 (2–9)
Olanzapine (10 mg)	50, 47	Neuropsychiatric Index	57.1	35.6	5 (2–64)
Olanzapine (15 mg)	53, 47	Neuropsychiatric Index	43.1	35.6	14 (4–∞)
Loxapine (10–50 mg)	19, 22	Clinical Global Impression mod-marked improvement	32	9	4 (2–∞)

Table 15 *continued.*

Drugs (dosage)	Number of patients (drug 1, placebo)	Measure BPSD	Drug 1 (%)	Drug 2 (%)	NNT (95%CI)
Haloperidol (2–10 mg)	20, 22	Clinical Global Impression mod-marked	35	9	4 (2–41)
Trifluoperazine (8 mg)	18, 9	Dementia and behavioural symptoms	22	0	5 (2–∞)
Tiapride (100–300 mg)	102, 101	MOSES	69	49	5 (3–15)
Haloperidol (3–6 mg)	99, 101	MOSES	63	49	7 (4–266)

Table 16 Numbers needed to harm (NNH) in placebo-controlled trials.

Drugs (mg)	Number of patients (drug 1, placebo)	Measure	Drug 1 (%)	Drug 2 (%)	NNH (95%CI)
Risperidone (0.25–4.0)	115, 114	EPSE	15	11	25 (8–∞)
Haloperidol (0.25–4.0)	115, 114	EPSE	22	11	9 (5–67)
Risperidone (0.25–4.0)	115, 114	Adverse events	76.5	72.8	27 (7–∞)
Haloperidol (0.25–4.0)	115, 114	Adverse events	80	72.8	14 (6–∞)
Risperidone (0.25–4.0)	115, 114	Somnolence	12.2	4.4	13 (7–139)
Haloperidol (0.25–4.0)	115, 114	Discontinuation	35.1	29.6	18 (6–∞)
Risperidone (0.25–4.0)	115, 114	Discontinuation	40.1	29.6	20 (4–∞)
Risperidone (1.0–2.0)	313, 163	Falls	19.2	20.2	100 (12–∞)
Risperidone (1.0–2.0)	313, 163	Somnolence	24	8	6 (4–11)
Risperidone (1.0–2.0)	313, 163	EPSE	17.3	7.4	10 (6–29)
Olanzapine (5)	56, 47	Discontinuation	19.6	23.4	33 (5–∞)
Olanzapine (10)	50, 47	Discontinuation	28	23.4	20 (4–∞)
Olanzapine (15)	53, 47	Discontinuation	34	23.4	9 (3–∞)

Table 16 *continued*.

Drugs (mg)	Number of patients (drug 1, placebo)	Measure	Drug 1 (%)	Drug 2 (%)	NNH (95%CI)
Olanzapine (5)	56, 47	Somnolence	20.4	6.4	7 (4–102)
Olanzapine (10)	50, 47	Somnolence	26	6.4	5 (3–17)
Olanzapine (15)	53, 47	Somnolence	35.8	6.4	3 (2–7)
Loxapine (0–50)	19, 22	Adverse events	90	55	3 (2–11)
Haloperidol (2–10)	20, 22	Adverse events	90	55	3 (2–10)
Trifluoperazine (8)	18, 9	Lethargy	61	0	2 (1–3)
Trifluoperazine (8)	18, 9	EPSE	44	0	2 (1–9)
Tiapride (100–300)	102, 101	Discontinuation	9.8	15.8	17 (7–∞)
Haloperidol (2–6)	99, 101	Discontinuation	21	15.8	20 (6–∞)
Tiapride (100–300)	102, 101	Discontinuation	15.7	17.5	56 (8–∞)
Haloperidol (2–6)	99, 101	Discontinuation	33.7	17.5	6 (4–23)

EPSE, extrapyramidal side effects.

particularly common with trifluoperazine 8 mg, loxapine 10–50 mg and haloperidol 2–10 mg. None of the trials found a significant rate of drop-out from the active treatment arm in comparison to the placebo.

Adverse effects in head to head anti-psychotic trials
The mortality rate in institutionalized patients in the trial that compared haloperidol 0.5–3 mg with trifluoperazine 1–6 mg was strikingly high (25% and 11% respectively).

Cholinesterase inhibitors

These are reviewed in detail in Chapter 7. Cholinesterase inhibitors lead to a delay or reduction in emergence of BPSDs or a decrease in the existing problem behaviours. These studies are mainly open label, single-agent studies and include only people with AD. Galantamine and donepezil, in particular, have both shown a significant reduction in BPSDs.

Anti-androgen drugs

There is a single report that suggests that medroxyprogesterone, a drug that lowers testosterone levels, may be effective in reducing inappropriate sexual behaviour in people with dementia.

Summary of practice recommendations in the use of drugs in BPSDs

For a summary, see *Box 30*.

Box 30 Practice recommendations for drug treatment of BPSD.

- Emergent BPSD symptoms should be investigated and any underlying pathology treated
- If the patient and carer are not distressed, pharmacological treatment is unnecessary
- Pharmacological treatment is only one element of management and should be used with and sometimes after other appropriate psychosocial measures
- Patients who are starting on cholinesterase inhibitors for cognitive effects should also have BPSD monitored and may require no other treatment
- Aggression and agitation may be treated with drugs that increase serotonin, which have fewer side effects than anti-psychotics; selective serotonin reuptake inhibitors (SSRIs) have the advantage of requiring only once daily dosage and so may be a first-line treatment
- Anticonvulsants are also effective but may need plasma levels monitoring and twice daily dosage
- Anti-psychotics are effective for a wider range of BPSD, although they have more side effects
- Naturalistic and randomized controlled trials (RCTs) suggest that low-dose olanzapine may be an effective and well-tolerated drug
- Low-dose risperidone and haloperidol are both cheaper and effective and tolerated in some patients; higher doses of both are more efficacious but less well tolerated
- Tiapride (a benzamide similar to sulpiride) also seem to be efficacious and well tolerated
- There are no RCTs on patients with dementia with Lewy bodies (DLB) but because of the lack of extrapyramidal side effects, quetiapine is the logical drug of choice

Delirium

Definition

Delirium (acute confusional state) is characterized by an acute onset of global but fluctuating disturbance of cognitive function, with disturbances in levels of consciousness – reduced clarity of awareness of the environment with reduced ability to focus, sustain or shift attention. This is usually accompanied by abnormalities in cognition, perception, mood and sleep–wake cycle. In most cases one or more specific organic causes can be identified.

Clinical features (Box 31)

Delirium frequently accompanies acute physical illness in older people and is an important trigger for psychiatric referral. It develops in up to 40% of hospitalized older people, in addition to about the 15% who have delirium on admission. Age and prior cognitive impairment are vulnerability factors for developing delirium. The most frequent presentation is of perplexity and sudden cognitive deterioration. Motor (tremor, mild ataxia) and autonomic abnormalities, such as sweating, tachycardia and postural hypotension, are common. Delirium can also present with acutely disturbed behaviour (e.g. pulling out intravenous lines or catheters) and verbal or physical aggression. Rapid changes in

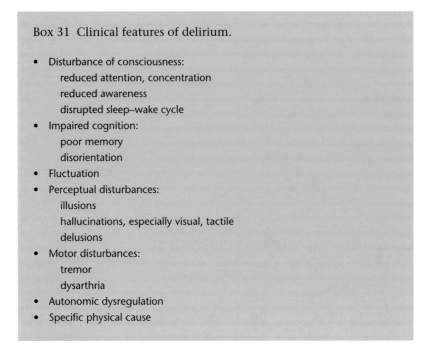

Box 31 Clinical features of delirium.

- Disturbance of consciousness:
  reduced attention, concentration
  reduced awareness
  disrupted sleep–wake cycle
- Impaired cognition:
  poor memory
  disorientation
- Fluctuation
- Perceptual disturbances:
  illusions
  hallucinations, especially visual, tactile
  delusions
- Motor disturbances:
  tremor
  dysarthria
- Autonomic dysregulation
- Specific physical cause

mental state and behaviour are often seen. Arousal may be heightened or alternatively reduced. Cognitive testing may reveal deficits in memory, attention, orientation and reasoning. Other mental state abnormalities may include altered perception, such as illusions (which may be very frightening). Visual and tactile hallucinations are also common. Intense but variable anxiety, perplexity and depression are common.

Differential diagnosis

Delirium may be difficult to distinguish from (often coexistent) dementia. Delirium should always be considered if a patient with an established dementia develops an acute deterioration in cognition or behaviour. Dementia with Lewy bodies (the characteristic features of which include vivid hallucinations and rapid fluctuation) often presents as a delirium with no apparent precipitating cause. Depression, mania and non-affective psychosis all have features in common with delirium but usually have a longer history and are not accompanied by altered consciousness.

Causes, risk factors and mechanisms

General
Delirium can be precipitated in older people by any major physical illness, or more minor illnesses in those who are vulnerable. Pre-existing visual impairment, cognitive deficits, severity of physical illness and dehydration are independent risk factors (*Box 32*). Common causes or precipitants (which are not mutually exclusive) are summarized in *Box 33*. No unifying mechanism for delirium has been identified. Factors implicated include increased blood–brain barrier permeability, impaired cholinergic neurotransmission and hypothalamic–pituitary axis dysregulation. Other neurotransmitters (particularly serotonin and dopamine) may also play a role.

Drug related (Box 34)
Age-related changes in drug handling increase the risk of toxicity of many drugs. Polypharmacy and relatively high dosage increase the risk further. Particular culprits include anticholinergic treatments for Parkinson's disease, antidepressants (especially tricyclic antidepressants with

---

Box 32 Risk factors.

- Pre-existing:
    visual impairment
    cognitive deficits
- Severity of physical illness
- Dehydration

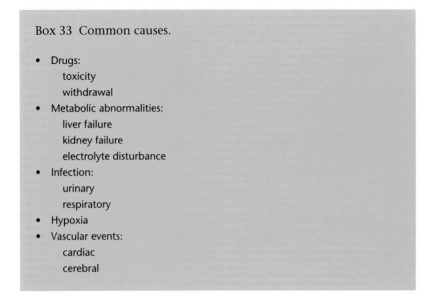

Box 33 Common causes.

- Drugs:
    toxicity
    withdrawal
- Metabolic abnormalities:
    liver failure
    kidney failure
    electrolyte disturbance
- Infection:
    urinary
    respiratory
- Hypoxia
- Vascular events:
    cardiac
    cerebral

Box 34 Drugs that commonly cause delirium.

- Anticholinergics
- Tricyclic antidepressants
- Trazodone
- Long-acting benzodiazepines
- Opioid analgesics
- Older anticonvulsants
- Quinolone antibiotics
- Diuretics
- Digoxin
- Typical anti-psychotics
- β Blockers
- Cimetidine

powerful anticholinergic effects, such as amitriptyline and trimipramine, and trazodone), long-acting benzodiazepines, opioid analgesics, older anticonvulsants, quinolone antibiotics, diuretics and digoxin. Other drugs commonly used in older people that carry a moderate risk of precipitating delirium include typical anti-psychotics, β blockers and cimetidine. Delirium may also be precipitated by withdrawal from alcohol or benzodiazepines and (less commonly) some selective serotonin reuptake inhibitors (SSRIs) (see Chapter 2). This may occur a few days after an acute hospital admission, when a patient has not given a history of alcohol misuse.

Outcome

Studies in acute hospital settings suggest that delirium is associated with increased length of inpatient care. About one patient in seven dies within a month of the onset of delirium. Of the remainder, nearly half require long-term residential care. Long-term risk of dementia is also increased.

Management

General principles

Ideally, delirium should be prevented; identification and close monitoring of medical patients at high risk are often effective. The main aims of assessment and management of established delirium are identification and treatment of underlying causes and exclusion of other conditions. Patients with apparent delirium require systematic assessment aimed at the identification of underlying causes and the exclusion of other conditions. A careful drug and substance misuse history is essential. Physical examination is particularly important, searching for evidence of specific systemic disease and of autonomic dysfunction. The most informative investigations are listed in *Box 35*).

The distress and behavioural disturbance complicating delirium may require symptomatic management and risk reduction pending response to definitive treatment. Physical restraint should be avoided wherever possible. Hydration and nutrition should be maintained, ample cues given to help maintain orientation including nursing in a well lit

Box 35 Informative investigations.

- Full blood count
- Erythrocyte sedimentation rate or C-reactive protein
- Urea and electrolytes
- Blood glucose
- Urinalysis and culture
- ECG
- Chest radiograph
- Pulse oximetry

environment and iatrogenic complications avoided. Falls and other injuries, dehydration and pressure sores are particular hazards. Delirium is often multifactorial; secondary maintaining factors such as anaemia, electrolyte disturbance and hypoxia should be identified and treated.

Drugs in the treatment of delirium
The most important aim is to reduce or stop drugs that might be causing or aggravating the delirium. Drugs may, however, be necessary and preferable to physical restraint in achieving behavioural control, reducing distress, and risk of injury or harm to self or others. There are no placebo-controlled trials of treatment for the behavioural and psychiatric symptoms of delirium. Anti-psychotics may be preferable to regular benzodiazepines, especially long acting benzodiazepines, the latter being more prone to cause worsening of confusion, oversedation, disinhibition and ataxia. Temazepam may, however, be used cautiously to help correct a disrupted sleep–wake cycle. Among the typical anti-psychotics, haloperidol is most widely used because of its relative lack of anticholinergic effects, liquid and injectable formulations and wide dose flexibility. It is, however, liable to cause extrapyramidal symptoms and a drop in blood pressure, both of which may lead to falls and immobility. In acute disturbance, a small dose of oral (if possible) or intramuscular lorazepam may be preferable to intramuscular haloperidol (0.5–1 mg). The minimum effective dose of haloperidol should be used, titrating up from

0.5 mg. Doses higher than 5 mg/day are seldom necessary. Clinicians should be absolutely clear that the patient does not have dementia with Lewy bodies (DLB) if prescribing haloperidol (see Chapter 7).

There is as yet little evidence supporting the use of atypical anti-psychotics, but first principles suggest that (as in dementia) their efficacy in achieving behavioural control will be similar to that of the typical anti-psychotics, although with a smaller side-effect burden. In general, doses should be as low as possible and similar to those used in dementia (see Chapter 7).

Treatment of delirium in the context of alcohol withdrawal

Acute alcohol withdrawal may cause a florid delirious state (delirium tremens), characterized by nausea and vomiting, tremor, sweating, headache, confusion, and vivid visual and tactile hallucinations. Anxiety and agitation are usually intense. Older people whose heavy drinking has not been suspected may be particularly vulnerable in the context of hospitalization for acute illness or for emergency or elective surgery. There is considerable risk of death or long-term morbidity, both second-ary to the delirium itself (within which electrolyte disturbance may be extreme, particularly if the patient is vomiting) and because of with-drawal fits and nutritional (particularly thiamine) deficiency. Both ben-zodiazepines and chlormethiazole are effective, with the former (usually diazepam or chlordiazepoxide) probably safer. Chlormethiazole has been associated with sudden death if the patient starts to drink again whilst taking it. The dose should be titrated rapidly down over 6–10 days, titrating the dose against severity of withdrawal symptoms. A typical regimen for an older person is shown in *Box 36*. Thiamine 200–300 mg daily or high-potency B vitamin complex should also be given for the first 3–5 days; the intramuscular route is usually used because the risk of anaphylaxis is minimized. Fits may require treatment with intravenous diazepam (Diazemuls 10 mg as necessary, infused slowly to lessen risk of respiratory depression). Metoclopramide 10 mg p.o. or i.m. every 6 hours is usually effective for vomiting. A long-term treatment plan should be formulated as soon as the patient is able to participate actively. The use of drugs in long-term treatment of alcohol dependence is limited. Disulfiram is seldom used in older people because of its toxicity in combination with alcohol. Both acamprosate and naltrexone are occasionally used. Their safety in older people has yet to be fully established. Both appear to be effective in reducing craving. Selective serotonin reuptake inhibitors (SSRIs) may be useful in reducing craving in older people with co-morbid depression and alcohol dependence.

Box 36 Typical alcohol withdrawal regimen.

- Days 1–3   Chlordiazepoxide 10 mg four times daily
- Days 4–5   5 mg four times daily
- Days 6–8   5 mg twice daily
- Days 9–10   2.5 mg twice daily

chapter 10

Psychotropics and drug interactions

There are several reasons why older people are at increased risk from drug interactions (*Box 37*). Both increasing age and the presence of mental health problems increase the likelihood that a patient will have significant physical problems. Older people with, for example, depression or dementia are in double jeopardy from a whole range of physical illnesses, particularly those affecting the cardiovascular and respiratory systems. The presence of a significant physical illness increases the chances that a patient will require treatment with drugs that might give rise to an adverse interaction if given together with drug treatment for the psychiatric condition. Such physical illness increases vulnerability to severe or irreversible consequences from any adverse drug interaction. Ageing is also associated with reduced levels of circulating binding proteins, particularly albumin. This tends to result in greater free concentrations of drugs that would otherwise be highly protein bound. Increasing age is also associated with marked changes in liver and kidney function. Both hepatic and renal blood flow are reduced in older people, and the activity of most liver enzymes also falls. Rates of first-pass metabolism, oxidation, reduction and hydrolysis are all reduced. Thus, both hepatic and renal clearance of many drugs are reduced. All these factors mean that there is a tendency towards increased circulating levels of many drugs for a given dose. There is, thereby, both a greater risk of side effects from drugs given alone and (more relevant to this chapter) an increased risk of adverse drug interactions.

Box 37 Age-related changes increasing risk of adverse drug interactions.

- Increased risk of:
    physical illness
    co-administered drugs
- Reduced levels of circulating binding proteins
- Greater free concentrations of protein-bound drugs
- Reduced hepatic and renal blood flow
- Reduced liver enzyme activity:
    first-pass metabolism
    oxidation
    reduction
    hydrolysis

The chapter focuses on those potential interactions that occur relatively frequently in clinical practice with older people and that carry clinically significant risk. In this context, it is important to consider which groups of drugs (other than psychotropics) older people are most likely to take, which include analgesics, antibiotics, antacids, anti-hypertensives, anticoagulants and anti-dysrhythmics.

The range of mechanisms that can result in adverse drug interactions is considered below. This is followed by a review of the specific interactions that older people are at risk of when taking each of the major groups of psychotropic drugs: the anti-psychotics (typical and atypical), the antidepressants (tricyclic, selective serotonin reuptake inhibitors (SSRIs) and other), the mood stabilizers, the hypnotics and analgesics, and the cholinesterase inhibitors.

Mechanisms of adverse interactions (Box 38)

Alterations in drug absorption are not often clinically important. However, antacids (which are often bought over the counter as well as being frequently prescribed) may reduce the absorption of benzodiazepines and thereby limit their sedative effect. This can result in increased benzodiazepine intake, leading in turn to exaggerated and harmful effects when the antacids are stopped. Altered renal clearance is more often relevant. The interaction between lithium and non-steroidal anti-inflammatory drugs (NSAIDs) is a good example. NSAIDs are of course another group of drugs frequently self or physician prescribed for older people. NSAID-induced reduction in prostaglandin synthesis causes reduced renal blood flow. This reduces excretion of lithium and, thus, increases blood lithium levels. High lithium levels are particularly hazardous in older people in whom the drug can cause neurotoxicity even at relatively low plasma levels. People with coexistent dementia or Parkinson's disease (both common in old age) are at particularly high risk.

Drug interactions may frequently be associated with changes in drug distribution. The co-administration of two drugs that are both extensively protein bound may result in higher free plasma levels of either or both. A good example of this is the potential for psychotropics that are very highly protein bound to displace co-administered warfarin, potentially causing excessive anticoagulation. This scenario is an increasingly important one, given the good evidence that warfarin protects older people with atrial fibrillation from suffering strokes.

When choosing an antidepressant or an anti-psychotic for a patient on warfarin, it is important to be aware of the differences in percentage protein binding between individual drugs in these groups. As far as anti-psychotics are concerned, clozapine and thioridazine are both very highly protein bound (95%), olanzapine and haloperidol almost as highly bound (93% and 92% respectively), whereas risperidone (88%)

Box 38 Mechanisms of adverse interaction.

- Absorption
- Renal clearance
- Distribution
- Metabolism

and quetiapine (83%) have a significantly higher free plasma fraction. Differences in percentage protein binding between SSRIs are more substantial. Sertraline is 99% protein bound, and fluoxetine and paroxetine 95% bound, but the other SSRIs have a much higher free plasma fraction – fluvoxamine is only 77% protein bound and citalopram only 50%.

Metabolic interactions may occur where concurrently administered drugs induce, inhibit or are metabolized by the same liver enzymes. Most such interactions involve cytochrome P450 subtypes. These liver enzymes exist in several genetically determined molecular forms. The growing science of psychopharmacogenomics is likely in the next few years to contribute very significantly to the prediction at individual level of both the likelihood of response to particular drugs and the vulnerability to adverse effects or interactions.

Drug interactions involving cytochrome P450 subtypes (Table 17)

A particular drug (psychotropic or otherwise) can affect the metabolism of another drug by *inhibiting* a cytochrome P450 (CYP450) subtype. Other drugs may influence its metabolism if it is a *substrate* for that particular hepatic metabolic pathway. Although more than 30 CYP450 coenzymes have been identified, these can be conveniently classified into four families: 2D6 (probably the most important in the context of psychotropic interactions), 1A2, 2C and 3A3/A4.

Cytochrome P450 2D6
A wide range of drugs is metabolized in part or wholly via CYP450 2D6. These include most tricyclic antidepressants and SSRIs, some other antidepressants (venlafaxine and nefazodone), some typical (haloperidol, thioridazine) and atypical (clozapine, risperidone, olanzapine) antipsychotics, the β blockers and some anti-arrhythmic drugs. The CYP450 2D6 system is significantly inhibited by fluphenazine and by many antidepressants, including moclobemide, nefazodone, mirtazapine and venlafaxine. Some SSRIs (including paroxetine, fluoxetine and its metabolite

Table 17 Cytochrome P450 subtypes: important substrates and inhibitors.

Subtype of cytochrome P450	Substrates	Inhibitors
2D6	TCAs	Paroxetine
	SSRIs	Fluoxetine (and norfluoxetine)
	Venlafaxine	Fluphenazine
	Nefazodone	Moclobemide
	Haloperidol	Nefazodone
	Thioridazine	Mirtazapine and venlafaxine
	Clozapine	Valproate
	Risperidone	
	Olanzapine	
	β Blockers	
	Anti-arrhythmic drugs	
2C	TCAs	Fluvoxamine
	Clozapine	Moclobemide
	Diazepam	Clozapine
	Phenytoin	Warfarin
	Omeprazole	
1A2	TCAs	Fluvoxamine
	Fluvoxamine	Mirtazapine
	Clozapine	Moclobemide
	Olanzapine	Olanzapine
	Tacrine	Cimetidine
	Paracetamol	
	Caffeine	
	Theophylline	
2C	TCAs	Fluvoxamine
	Clozapine	Moclobemide
	Diazepam	Clozapine
	Phenytoin	
	Omeprazole	
	Warfarin	
3A3/4	TCAs	Ketoconazole
	Atypical anti-psychotics	Nefazodone
	Carbamazepine	SSRIs (except citalopram)
	Alprazolam	Mirtazapine
	Triazolam	
	Calcium channel blockers	
	Terfenadine	
	Astemizole	

SSRIs, selective serotonin reuptake inhibitors; TCAs, tricyclic antidepressants.

norfluoxetine, and sertraline) are particularly powerful inhibitors of CYP450 2D6.

The potential for adverse drug interactions involving the cytochrome P450 2D6 system is highest in the subgroup of the population (approximately 7%) who have a genetically determined low level of 2D6 activity.

Cytochrome P450 1A2

Approximately 12% of the population show low levels of activity of CYP450 1A2. Drugs extensively metabolized by this pathway include the tricyclic antidepressants and the SSRI fluvoxamine, the atypical anti-psychotics clozapine and olanzapine, the cholinesterase inhibitor tacrine, and a number of non-psychotropic drugs including paracetamol, caffeine and theophylline. CYP450 1A2 activity is inhibited most markedly by fluvoxamine, and also by other antidepressants (mirtazapine and moclobemide), the atypical anti-psychotic olanzapine and the histamine H_2-receptor antagonist cimetidine.

Cytochrome P450 2C

Cytochrome P450 2C is particularly important in the 2% of white people and 20% of Japanese people who are relatively poor metabolizers via this route. The main substrates for this enzyme family are the tricyclic antidepressants, the atypical anti-psychotic clozapine, diazepam, phenytoin, omeprazole and warfarin. CYP450 2C is significantly inhibited by the antidepressants fluvoxamine and moclobemide and by clozapine.

Cytochrome P450 3A3/A4

Cytochrome P450 3A3/A4 has a wide range of both psychotropic and non-psychotropic substrates. These include tricyclic antidepressants, atypical anti-psychotics, carbamazepine, alprazolam and triazolam, calcium channel blockers, and the antihistamines terfenadine and astemizole. It is most powerfully inhibited by the antifungal agent ketoconazole. This may have particular relevance in psychiatry because of the possible use of this drug (which dramatically reduces cortisol levels) in refractory depression. CYP450 3A/4 is also significantly inhibited by nefazodone, by all SSRIs (particularly fluvoxamine and fluoxetine) except citalopram, and by mirtazapine.

Pharmacodynamic interactions may be very hazardous. An example of such an interaction is the combination of monoamine oxidase inhibitors (MAOIs) and antidepressants that block serotonin reuptake, which can result in dramatic increases in serotonin levels and cause a (potentially fatal) 'serotonin syndrome'. This syndrome and its range of possible drug interaction-related causes are discussed in more detail below.

The serotonin syndrome (Table 18)

The serotonin syndrome is a dangerous and potentially fatal condition that may be induced by serotoninergic enhancers, particularly if these are taken in combination. Serotoninergic enhancers include not only the SSRIs and MAOIs but also some tricyclic antidepressants (particularly clomipramine), L-tryptophan, lithium, carbamazepine, some opiates, buspirone and the triptans (e.g. sumatriptan), which are increasingly being used in the treatment of migraine. Hypertension and atherosclerosis (both age-related conditions) also appear to be risk factors for the serotonin syndrome. The serotonin syndrome is characterized by a range of cognitive–behavioural, autonomic and neuromuscular abnormalities. The cognitive–behavioural changes include confusion, agitation, elation

Table 18 The serotonin syndrome.

Cognitive–behavioural	Autonomic	Neuromuscular
Confusion	Gastrointestinal disturbance:	Clumsiness
Agitation	nausea	Incoordination
Elation	vomiting	Tremor
Irritability	diarrhoea	Increased tone
	fever	Hyperreflexia
	Labile blood pressure	

and/or irritability. The syndrome should therefore be considered in the differential diagnosis of apparent mania. Autonomic aspects of the syndrome include gastrointestinal disturbance (nausea, vomiting, diarrhoea), fever and marked changes in blood pressure. Neuromuscular abnormalities include clumsiness and incoordination, tremor, increased tone and hyperreflexia. A serotonin syndrome should be suspected in an older person who develops any of these clinical features while taking one or (especially) more than one serotoninergic enhancer.

Conclusions

The drugs which have adverse interactions with antidepressants, mood stabilizers, antipsychotics and cholinesterase inhibitors are summarized in Tables 19, 20, 21, 22, respectively. Older people are at particular risk of adverse drug interactions because of their higher rate of multisystem morbidity and their increased likelihood of receiving polypharmacy. Age-related changes in drug handling also increase the risk of adverse interactions.

The strongest evidence in the literature for relevant interactions in older people reflects changes in renal excretion (particularly relevant for lithium) and cytochrome P450 (relevant for a wide range of psychotropic and other drugs). Awareness of potential interactions is an important component of safe prescribing practice for older people with mental health problems.

Table 19 Adverse interactions with antidepressants.

Drug/class	Possible adverse interaction with	Comments
TCAs	Anticholinergics	Additive anticholinergic effects can cause ileus, hypothermia
	Alcohol, sympathomimetics	Additive toxicity
	SSRIs and other serotonin enhancers	Serotonin syndrome
	Carbamazepine	Cardiotoxicity
	Lithium	Tremor
SSRIs	Drugs metabolized via cytochrome P450 subtypes	See Table 17
	Warfarin	Monitor anticoagulation closely
	Carbamazepine	Increased carbamazepine toxicity
SSRIs, venlafaxine, nefazodone	MAOIs	**Avoid!!**
Fluoxetine, fluvoxamine	Theophylline	Theophylline toxicity
Fluvoxamine	Terfenadine, astemizole	Increased antihistamine toxicity
	Tacrine	Increased tacrine toxicity
MAOIs	SSRIs, venlafaxine, nefazodone, reboxetine, opiates, sympathomimetics	**Avoid**
Moclobemide	As for MAOIs except opiates	Relatively safe with morphine, diamorphine
	Lithium, TCAs and sumatriptan	Caution

MAOIs, monoamine oxidase inhibitors; SSRIs, selective serotonin reuptake inhibitors; TCAs, tricyclic antidepressants.

Table 20 Adverse interactions with mood stabilizers.

Drug/class	Possible adverse interaction with	Comments
Lithium	ACE inhibitors, diuretics, NSAIDs	Increased lithium toxicity
	Verapamil	Neurotoxicity, bradycardia
	Phenothiazines, haloperidol	Neurotoxicity
Carbamazepine	Fluoxetine, fluvoxamine, cimetidine, dextropropoxyphene	Carbamazepine toxicity
	Warfarin	Reduced anticoagulation

ACE, angiotensin-converting enzyme; NSAIDs, non-steroidal anti-inflammatory drugs.

Table 21 Adverse interactions with anti-psychotics.

Drug/class	Possible adverse interaction with	Comments
Phenothiazines	Cimetidine	Increased sedation
All typical anti-psychotics	Dopamine enhancers/ inhibitors	Increased extrapyramidal effects
Haloperidol	Fluoxetine	Increased extrapyramidal effects
	Terfenadine, astemizole	Increased antihistamine toxicity
Pimozide	Cardioactive drugs, diuretics	Cardiotoxicity
Clozapine	Fluvoxamine, fluoxetine	Increased clozapine toxicity
	Cytotoxics, sulphonamides, chloramphenicol	Increased risk of blood dyscrasias
	Lithium	Neurotoxicity
	Benzodiazepines	Sedation, respiratory depression
Quetiapine, risperidone	SSRIs	Increased anti-psychotic levels
Quetiapine	Nefazodone, ketoconazole	Increased anti-psychotic levels
Olanzapine	Fluvoxamine	Increased anti-psychotic levels
Zotepine	Diazepam, fluoxetine	Increased anti-psychotic levels
Ziprazidone	Cimetidine	Increased anti-psychotic levels
	Carbamazepine	Decreased anti-psychotic levels

SSRIs, selective serotonin reuptake inhibitors.

Table 22 Adverse interactions with cholinesterase inhibitors.

Drug/class	Possible adverse interaction with	Comments
Donepezil, galantamine	Fluvoxamine, ketoconazole	Increased cholinergic side effects

References and further reading

References

Klysner R, Bent-Hantsen J, Hansen HL et al. Efficacy of citalopram in the prevention of recurrent depression in elderly patients: placebo-controlled study of maintenance therapy. *Br J Psych* 2002; **181**: 29–35

Nair NP, Amin M, Holm P et al, Moclobemide and nortryptyline in elderly depressed patients: a randomized multicentre trial against placebo. *J Affect Dis* 1995; **33**: 1–9

Nyth AL, Gottfries CG, Lyby K et al, A controlled multicentre study of placebo and citalopram in elderly depressed patients with and without concomitant dementia. *Acta Psychiatr Scand* 1992; **86**: 138–45

Pampallona S, Bollini P, Tibaldi G, Kupelnick B, Munizza C, Patient compliance in the treatment of depression. *Br J Psychiatry* 2002; **180**: 104–9

Tollefson GD, Bosomworth JC, Heiligenstein JH et al, A double-blind, placebo-controlled clinical trial of fluoxetine in geriatric patients with major depression. *Int Psychogeriatrics* 1995; **7**: 89–104

Wakelin JS, Fluvoxamine in the treatment of the older depressed patient; double-blind, placebo-controlled. *Int Clin Psychopharm* 1986; **1**: 221–30

Further reading

Alexopoulos GS, Abrams RC, Young RC, Shamoian CA, Cornell Scale for depression in dementia. *Biol Psychiatry* 1988; **23**: 271–84

Altman DG, Confidence intervals for the number needed to treat. *BMJ* 1998; **317**: 1309–12

American Psychiatric Association, *Diagnostic and Statistical Manual of Mental Disorders – IV*. Washington DC: American Psychiatric Association, 1987

Beekman ATF, Copeland JRM, Prince MJ, Review of community prevalence of depression in late life. *Br J Psychiatry* 1999; **174**: 307–11

Birks JS, Melzer D, Beppu H, Donepezil for mild and moderate Alzheimer's disease (Cochrane Review). In: *The Cochrane Library*, Issue 1. Oxford: Update Software, 2002

Britton A, Russell R, Multidisciplinary team interventions for delirium in patients with chronic cognitive impairment (Cochrane Review). In: *The Cochrane Library*, Issue 1. Oxford: Update Software, 2002

Cook RJ, Sackett DL, The number needed to treat: a clinically useful measure of treatment effect. *BMJ* 1995; **310**: 452–4

Fahy M, Livingston G (2002) A systematic review of the outcome of antipsychotic treatment in older people with dementia: a number needed to treat analysis. Submitted

Hoyl MT, Alessi CA, Harker JO et al, Development and testing of a five item version of the Geriatric Depression Scale. *J Am Geriatr Soc* 1999; **47**: 873–8

Jacoby R, Oppenheimer C, *Psychiatry and the Elderly*, 3rd edn. Oxford: Oxford University Press, 2001

Katona C, Livingston G, How well do antidepressants work in older people? A systematic review of number needed to treat. *J Affect Disord* 2002; **69**: 47–52.

Kirchner V, Kelly CA, Harvey RJ, Thioridazine for dementia (Cochrane Review). In: *The Cochrane Library*, Issue 1. Oxford: Update Software, 2002

Lindesay J (ed), *Neurotic Disorders in the Elderly*, Vol. 10. Oxford: Oxford University Press, 1995

Livingston G, Katona C, How useful are cholinesterase inhibitors in the treatment of Alzheimer's disease? a number needed to treat analysis. *Int J Geriatr Psychiatry* 2000; **15**: 203–7

Livingston G, Watkin V, Milne B, Manela M, Katona C, The natural history of depression and the anxiety disorders in older people. *J Affect Dis* 1997; **46**: 255–62

Lonergan E, Luxenberg J, Colford J, Haloperidol for agitation in dementia (Cochrane Review). In: *The Cochrane Library*, Issue 1. Oxford: Update Software, 2002

Mittmann N, Herrmann N, Einarson TR et al, The efficacy, safety and tolerability of antidepressants in late life depression: a meta-analysis. *J Affect Dis* 1997; **46**: 191–217

Pampallona S, Bollini P, Tibaldi G, Kupelnick B, Munizza C, Patient compliance in the treatment of depression. *Br J Psychiatry* 2002; **180**: 104–9

Taylor D, McConnell H, Duncan-McConnell, Kerwin R, *The South London and Maudsley Prescribing Guidelines 2001 Prescribing Guidelines*, 6th edn. London: Martin Dunitz, 2001

Williams PS, Rands G, Orrell M, Spector A, Aspirin for vascular dementia (Cochrane Review). In: *The Cochrane Library*, Issue 4. Oxford: Update Software, 2001

Wilson K, Mottram P, Sivanranthan A, Nightingale A, Antidepressants versus placebo for the depressed elderly (Cochrane Review). In: *The Cochrane Library*, Issue 4. Oxford: Update Software, 2001

World Health Organization, *International Classification of Mental Disorders*, 10th edn. Geneva: World Health Organization, 1992

Index